Workbook for use with

Medical Insurance

An Integrated Claims Process Approach

Sixth Edition

Joanne D. Valerius, MPH, RHIA
Director, Health Information Management Certificate Program, Oregon Health and Science University

Nenna L. Bayes, BBA, MEd
Professor, Program Coordinator of Office Systems Administration, Ashland Community and Technical College

Cynthia Newby, CPC, CPC-P

Amy L. Blochowiak, MBA, ACS, AIAA, AIRC, ARA, FLHC, FLMI, HCSA, HIA, HIPAA, MHP, PCS, SILA-F
Northeast Wisconsin Technical College

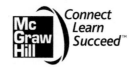

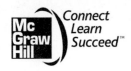

The McGraw-Hill Companies

Connect
Learn
Succeed™

WORKBOOK FOR USE WITH MEDICAL INSURANCE: AN INTEGRATED CLAIMS
PROCESS APPROACH, SIXTH EDITION
JOANNE D. VALERIUS, NENNA L. BAYES, CYNTHIA NEWBY,
AND AMY L. BLOCHOWIAK

Published by McGraw-Hill, a business unit of The McGraw-Hill Companies, Inc., 1221
Avenue of the Americas, New York, NY 10020. Copyright © 2014 by The McGraw-Hill
Companies, Inc. All rights reserved. Printed in the United States of America. Previous
editions © 2002, 2005, 2008, 2010, and 2012.

The contents, or parts thereof, may be reproduced in print form solely for classroom use with
Medical Insurance: An Integrated Claims Process Approach, Sixth Edition, provided such
reproductions bear copyright notice, but may not be reproduced in any other form or for any
other purpose without the prior written consent of The McGraw-Hill Companies, Inc.,
including, but not limited to, in any network or other electronic storage or transmission, or
broadcast for distance learning.

1 2 3 4 5 6 7 8 9 0 QDB/QDB 1 0 9 8 7 6 5 4 3

ISBN 978-0-07-752051-9
MHID 0-07-752051-3

All brand or product names are trademarks or registered trademarks of their respective
companies.

CPT five-digit codes, nomenclature, and other data are © 2012 American Medical
Association. All rights reserved. No fee schedules, basic unit, relative values, or related
listings are included in the CPT. The AMA assumes no liability for the data contained herein.

CPT codes are based on CPT 2013.
ICD-10-CM codes are based on ICD-10-CM 2013

All names, situations, and anecdotes are fictitious. They do not represent any person, event,
or medical record.

www.mhhe.com

Table of Contents

Preface iv

PART 1   **WORKING WITH MEDICAL INSURANCE AND BILLING**

Chapter 1   Introduction to the Medical Billing Cycle 1

Chapter 2   Electronic Health Records, HIPAA, and HITECH:
               Sharing and Protecting Patients' Health Information 21

Chapter 3   Patient Encounters and Billing Information 35

PART 2   **CLAIM CODING**

Chapter 4   Diagnostic Coding: ICD-10-CM 49

Chapter 5   Procedural Coding: CPT AND HCPCS 62

Chapter 6   Visit Charges and Compliant Billing 84

PART 3   **CLAIMS**

Chapter 7   Health Care Claim Preparation and Transmission 97

Chapter 8   Private Payers/BlueCross BlueShield 108

Chapter 9   Medicare 122

Chapter 10   Medicaid 136

Chapter 11   TRICARE and CHAMPVA 144

Chapter 12   Workers' Compensation and Disability/Automotive Insurance 153

PART 4   **CLAIM FOLLOW-UP AND PAYMENT PROCESSING**

Chapter 13   Payments (RAs), Appeals, and Secondary Claims 164

Chapter 14   Patient Billing and Collections 179

Note to Students: Chapter 15-Primary Case Studies and Chapter 16-RA/Secondary Case Studies in the main *Medical Insurance, 6e* text are not covered in the workbook.

PART 5   **HOSPITAL SERVICES**

Chapter 17   Hospital Billing and Reimbursement 191

               Forms 201

Preface

The *Workbook for use with Medical Insurance,* 6e, is intended to strengthen, reinforce, and expand student learning of the skills and concepts presented in the text. This workbook complements the text and follows the same learning outcomes as *Medical Insurance,* 6e. The workbook has been updated to reflect the changes in the main text. For a detailed list of changes, please refer to the Preface in *Medical Insurance, 6e.*

Workbook chapters include a brief review of the math skills necessary for processing medical insurance claims where applicable. Reinforcement of reading assignments (or note taking) is easy for students following the Assisted Outlining activity. The key terms activities help strengthen students' vocabulary for each chapter, and the Applying Concepts activities provide additional hands-on practice with the concepts and skills presented in each chapter.

Instructors can measure each student's progress using the Self-Quiz and Critical Thinking questions. Instructors can also expand on the web activities to deepen student understanding or to introduce new topics, for instance, when private and governmental third-party providers' policies change.

For classes that are one semester in length, it is suggested that the workbook materials be used as homework assignments for reinforcement, follow-up, or extra instruction. For classes longer than one semester, the workbook materials can be used in class as well as for homework assignments. Additional class time would also provide the opportunity to have students work in teams or groups on several of the Internet exercises.

Instructors may choose to use sections of the workbook in class, for example, using the key terms section as a pretest. Instructors may select individual assignments for each chapter depending on the progress of the class or assign specific activities to students who might be having difficulty grasping certain themes. For example, the instructor might assign all students the Assisted Outlining activity to reinforce the reading of each chapter, or the Self-Quiz questions could be used by students individually or as a class as a pretest before chapter or part tests.

Other students may need critical thinking skills sharpened or wish to focus on one of the Internet activities, Using the Web Wisely and Web Scavenger Hunt. The additional activities could be used in their entirety, or portions may be selected to highlight individual concepts from the text.

The *Instructor's Manual for use with Medical Insurance,* 6e, provides keys to all activities, including the answers to the Assisted Outlining activities. Instructors can access the Instructor's Manual via the book's Online Learning Center website, www.mhhe.com/valerius6e.

ACKNOWLEDGMENTS

Thanks to the instructors and reviewers who have provided feedback on the workbook's different editions. A full list of reviewers can be found in the Acknowledgments section of the main text, *Medical Insurance, 6e.*

TO THE STUDENT

Welcome to the world of health care. This workbook is designed to help you prepare for your career as a medical billing specialist, an integral part of providing quality health care to patients. This workbook, which accompanies your *Medical Insurance,* 6e text, is intended to help you strengthen, reinforce, and expand your learning of the skills and concepts presented in the text.

For maximum results, we suggest that you complete the Assisted Outlining activity for each chapter. This reinforces what you have read in the textbook and gives you an opportunity to take notes on the textbook material.

To improve or expand your medical vocabulary, focus on the key terms; these exercises can also be used as a pretest. Other workbook activities focus on applying what you have learned in the text and class. There are many Self-Quiz and Critical Thinking questions to help you assess what you have mastered and what you still need to study. Web activities allow you to step-up your learning on various topics. Included for your use at the end of Chapters 1 and 3 are brief reviews of the math skills necessary for processing medical insurance claims. Study these reviews if you need to go over the math before answering the Applying Concepts questions.

OUTLINE

Following is a brief outline of the text and the workbook.

Part	Coverage
1: Working with Medical Insurance and Billing	Covers Steps 1 through 3 of the medical billing cycle by introducing the major types of medical insurance, payers, and regulators, as well as the medical billing cycle. Also covers HIPAA/HITECH Privacy, Security, and Electronic Healthcare Transactions/Code Sets, and Breach Notification rules.
2: Claim Coding	Covers Steps 4 through 6 of the medical billing cycle, while building skills in correct coding procedures, use of coding references, and compliance with proper linkage guidelines.
3: Claims	Covers Step 7 of the medical billing cycle by covering the general procedures for calculating reimbursement, how to bill compliantly, and preparing and transmitting claims.
4: Claim Follow-up and Payment Processing	Covers Steps 8 through 10 of the medical billing cycle by providing descriptions of the major third-party private and government-sponsored payers' procedures and regulations, along with specific filing guidelines. Also explains how to handle payments from payers, follow up and appeal claims, file secondary claims, and correctly bill and collect from patients. This part includes two case studies chapters that provide exercises to reinforce knowledge of completing primary/secondary claims, processing payments from payers, and handling patients' accounts. These case studies, in the main text, can be completed via simulated Medisoft V17 exercises available in McGraw-Hill's online homework management system, *Connect Plus*.
5: Hospital Services	Provides necessary background in hospital billing, coding, and payment methods.

Please note that this workbook contains no activities corresponding to Chapters 15 and 16 in the main text, *Medical Insurance*, 6e, because they are case studies chapters.

—The authors

Chapter 1 Introduction to the Medical Billing Cycle

Learning Outcomes

After studying this chapter, you should be able to:

1.1 Identify three ways that medical insurance specialists help ensure the financial success of physician practices.

1.2 Differentiate between covered and noncovered services under medical insurance policies.

1.3 Compare indemnity and managed care approaches to health plan organization.

1.4 Discuss three examples of cost containment employed by health maintenance organizations.

1.5 Explain how a preferred provider organization works.

1.6 Describe the two elements that are combined in a consumer-driven health plan.

1.7 Define the three major types of medical insurance payers.

1.8 Explain the ten steps in the medical billing cycle.

1.9 Analyze how professionalism and etiquette contribute to career success.

1.10 Evaluate the importance of professional certification for career advancement.

ASSISTED OUTLINING

Directions: *Read the chapter through one time. Then go back over the chapter and find the information required to complete the following outline of the chapter. Write the requested information directly in the spaces provided.*

Administrative staff members help collect the maximum appropriate payments by:

1.

2.

3.

1.1 Working in the Medical Insurance Field

Rising Spending on Health Care

1. The foremost factor contributing to the increased costs of health care is:

2. Why is it important to manage the business side of a physician practice?

Administrative Complexity Increases Opportunities

3. With how many health plans does the average practice work?

Helping to Ensure Financial Success

4. What does it mean to manage cash flow?

Following Procedures

5. Who commonly heads administrative staff?

Communicating

6. What skills do effective communicators possess?

Using Health Information Technology

7. Name three types of health information technology (HIT).

   (1)   **(3)**

   (2)

A Note of Caution: What Health Information Technology Cannot Do

8. Computers are not more accurate than the _____ who is entering the data.

1.2 Medical Insurance Basics

1. Medical insurance is an agreement between a _____ and a _____.

Health Care Benefits

2. A medically _____ service is both reasonable and consistent with standards for the diagnosis or treatment of injury or illness.

Covered Services

3. Annual physical examinations, immunizations, and routine screening procedures are _____ medical services.

Noncovered Services

4. What is the difference between a covered service and a noncovered service?

5. List four typical noncovered services:

(1)   (3)

(2)   (4)

Group or Individual Medical Insurance Policies

6. Which generally costs the policyholder less, a group or an individual policy?

Disability/Automotive Insurance and Workers' Compensation

7. Disability insurance covers income lost because a person cannot

_____ .

8. Workers' compensation covers _____-related accidents.

1.3 Health Care Plans

What are the two types of health care plans?

1.

2.

Indemnity

Conditions for Payment

3. What four conditions must be met before the insurance company makes a payment for an indemnity claim?

(1)   (3)

(2)   (4)

Fee-for-Service Payment Approach

4. Is a fee-for-service payment made before or after services are provided?_____

Managed Care

5. List the four basic types of managed care plans:

(1)   (3)

(2)   (4)

1.4 Health Maintenance Organizations

1. HMOs have _____ of physicians, hospitals, and other providers.

2. Is a capitation payment made before or after services are provided?_____

3. What five methods does an HMO use to contain costs?

    (1)   (4)

    (2)   (5)

    (3)

4. The health care quality improvements made by HMOs are illustrated by (1) _____ and (2) _____.

Point-of-Service Plans

5. A point-of-service plan is also called an _____ HMO.

1.5 Preferred Provider Organizations

1. Which type of plan is more popular, the HMOs or the PPOs?_____

1.6 Consumer-Driven Health Plans

1. What are the two elements of a consumer-directed health plan (CDHP)?

    (1)

    (2)

1.7 Medical Insurance Payers

Medical insurance payers are categorized into three groups. They are:

1.

2.

3.

Private Payers

4. Private payers include the large _____ companies.

Self-Funded Health Plans

5. A self-funded health plan insures _____ instead of paying premiums to an insurance carrier.

Government-Sponsored Health Care Programs

The four major government-sponsored health care programs and the populations they serve are:

6.

7.

8.

9.

1.8 The Medical Billing Cycle

Medical insurance specialists handle the administrative work that is part of the payment process. What do these functions entail?

1.

2.

3.

4.

5.

6.

7.

8.

9.

10.

These functions are organized under the medical billing cycle. List, in order, the steps in this cycle.

Step 1

Step 2

Step 3

Step 4

Step 5

Step 6

Step 7

Step 8

Step 9

Step 10

1.9 Achieving Success

Medical insurance specialists work in (list at least five):

1.

2.

3.

4.

5.

Requirements for Success

What are the skills and attributes of successful medical insurance specialists?

Skills

6.

7.

8.

9.

10.

11.

12.

Attributes

13.

14.

15.

16.

Medical Ethics and Etiquette in the Practice

17. Explain the difference between medical ethics and professional etiquette.

1.10 Moving Ahead

What are some ways to secure a medical insurance specialist position or advance on the job? (List at least three.)

1.

2.

3.

What are the benefits of achieving a professional certification?

4.

KEY TERMS

Multiple Choice

Circle the letter of the choice that best matches the definition or answers the question.

1. A list of the medical services covered by an insurance policy.

   A. Health care claim
   B. Schedule of benefits
   C. Noncovered services
   D. Fee-for-service

2. Health plans are often referred to as:

   A. Policyholders
   B. Subscribers
   C. Providers
   D. Payers

3. A managed care network of providers under contract to provide services at discounted fees.

   A. Health Maintenance Organization (HMO)
   B. Preferred Provider Organization (PPO)
   C. Point-of-Service Plan (POS)
   D. Open-access plan

4. A fixed prepayment made to a medical provider for all necessary, contracted services provided to each patient who is a plan member for a specific period.

   A. Capitation
   B. Benefit
   C. Participation
   D. Payer

5. A health plan that reimburses based on the fees charged.

   A. Indemnity
   B. PPO
   C. Managed care
   D. Disability

6. An amount that a health plan requires a beneficiary to pay at the time of service for each health care encounter.

   A. Deductible
   B. Copayment
   C. Coinsurance
   D. Fee-for-service

7. A percentage of each charge that an insured person must pay.

    A. Deductible   **C.** Coinsurance

    B. Copayment   **D.** Fee-for-service

8. A practice's operating expenses.

    A. Cash flow   **C.** Accounts receivable (AR)

    B. PM/EHR   **D.** Accounts payable (AP)

9. A health plan that combines a health plan, usually a managed care plan, and a "savings account" used to pay medical bills before the deductible has been met.

    A. MSA   **C.** CDHP

    B. PPO   **D.** HMO

10. Payments for medical services.

    A. Fee-for-services   **C.** Benefits

    B. Capitation   **D.** Third-party payer

SELF-QUIZ

1. Who are the three participants in the medical insurance relationship?

2. The key to coverage is medical necessity. How is this term defined?

3. When and how is a fee-for-service paid?

4. When is capitation paid?

5. Medical insurance, which is also known as health insurance, is a written contract between which two parties?

6. The policyholder, also called the insured or the member, pays a premium. In exchange, the health plan provides _____.

7. Benefits usually are defined as:

8. Covered services are those shown on _____.

9. A managed care plan's goals are:

10. Capitation is derived from what language? _____ Meaning? _____

11. What is the definition of capitation?

12. How are charges paid in the capitated rate payment system?

13. Name the three main job functions of medical insurance specialists.

14. Practice management programs (PMPs) are used for _____.

15. Medical insurance specialists are employed in (list five).

(1) _____

(2) _____

(3) _____

(4) _____

(5) _____

CRITICAL THINKING QUESTIONS

1. Should preexisting conditions be covered? Why or why not?

2. For you, which would be the preferred health insurance plan? Indemnity or managed care? Why?

3. Of the managed care health plans, which plan is right for you?

4. If you were a practice manager, how would you evaluate the benefits and disadvantages of fee-for-service compared with capitated plans?

5. There are many skills/attributes that the medical insurance specialist possesses. Identify those skills/attributes that you already possess and those that you need to work on.

WEB ACTIVITIES

Surfing the Net

1. Using a search engine such as Google or Yahoo, locate the website of an indemnity insurer in your state/region/city.

    A. What types of policies/plans are offered by this company?

    _____

    _____

    B. Can individuals purchase policies from this company?

    _____

    _____

    C. Does this company offer insurance plans in other states?

    _____

    _____

    D. Is this insurer associated with the Blue Cross or Blue Shield organizations?

    _____

    _____

    _____

    E. From the website:
        1. Can you discover what services are covered and what services are not covered under this health plan?

        _____

        _____

        2. Are preexisting conditions covered?

        _____

        _____

        3. Can you determine the cost of purchasing a policy?

        _____

        _____

2. Using a search engine such as Google or Yahoo, locate the website of another health care insurer in your state/region/city.

    A. Does this company only offer indemnity policies?

    _____

    _____

    B. Is this insurer associated with the Blue Cross or Blue Shield organizations?

    _____

    _____

3. Using the same search engine, locate a website of a managed care insurer in your state/community.

    A. Does this company offer more than one type of plan?

    _____

    _____

B. What is the copayment for each plan?

_____

_____

C. Do physicians in your area contract with this plan?

_____

_____

D. Do hospitals in your area contract with this plan?

_____

_____

Using the Web Wisely

Using a search engine such as Google or Yahoo, locate the website of the Medical Billing Advocates of America.

4. Authority
   - Is the author identified?

   _____

   - Credentials?

   _____

   - Can you verify?

   _____

   _____

5. Purpose and coverage
   - What is the address extension? .com, .edu, .gov, .org?

   _____

   - Can you identify the purpose? What is it?

   _____

   - Can you identify the depth of coverage?
       - Comprehensive?
       - Narrow?

   _____

   _____

6. Accuracy
   - Is the page edited or reviewed by outside specialists?

   _____

   - Are the facts correct and references cited?

   _____

   - Based on your level of knowledge, does it seem credible?

   _____

7. Timeliness
   • When was the site created?

   _____

   • When was the site last updated?

   _____

8. Integrity of the information
   • Are sources clearly labeled?

   _____

   • Are references clearly cited?

   _____

   • If pictures are used to convey information, could they have been digitally enhanced/edited?

   _____

9. Objectivity or point of view
   • Does a particular point of view come across?

   _____

   • Does the site use inflammatory or provocative language?

   _____

   • If there are ads on the page, are they easily differentiated from the actual page?

   _____

   • Is there a connection between the advertisements and the webpage?

   _____

WEB SCAVENGER HUNT

Using a search engine such as Google or Yahoo, can you find a certification for medical billers? Medical coders? Medical office managers? Explore these sites, using the questions posed to determine if one of these certifications is right for you.

USING MATH IN THE MEDICAL OFFICE

Proper calculation of patient statements is an essential part of the medical insurance specialist's job. Calculating the amounts billed to and reimbursed from payers is equally important. Let's start with a quick review of math in the medical office.

Per cent originated with Latin words that mean "out of 100." When you state a percentage, you are saying the same thing as "80 out of every 100 doctors belong to a professional organization," or "80 percent of doctors belong to a professional organization." We also use the percent symbol (%) to indicate percents, or "80% of doctors belong to a professional organization."

CHANGING PERCENTS TO DECIMALS

Moving Decimals

To calculate a percentage of a number, rewrite the percentage as a decimal. This is easy to do by moving the decimal point two (2) places to the left. For example, to write 80 percent as a decimal:

$$80\% = .80$$

To write 67.5 percent as a decimal:

$$67.5\% = .675$$

Dividing by 100

Moving the decimal point two places to the left is also the same as dividing the number by 100. For example, to change 80 percent to a decimal:

$$80 \div 100 = .80$$

To change 67.5 percent to a decimal:

$$67.5 \div 100 = .675$$

Exercise 1

Change these percentages to decimals. Try using both methods of changing percentages to decimals.

A. 75%

B. 25.3%

C. 47%

D. 88.5%

E. 07%

Finding the Percentage

Now multiply the decimal number by the number for which you are seeking a percentage. The result is the percentage.

$$.80 \times 100 = 80$$

Imagine ordering 100 tongue depressors to use in the medical office. Upon receiving the order, the office supply company responds saying only 57 percent of the tongue depressors can be delivered today. First, find the decimal equivalent of 57 percent. Next, multiply the decimal by 100.

$$57\% = .57 \qquad \text{OR} \qquad 57 \div 100 = .57$$

$$.57 \times 100 = 57$$

Of the 100 tongue depressors ordered, only 57 will be delivered today.

Exercise 2

Needless to say, not all percentages are calculated using a total of 100. For example, practice finding these percentages.

A. 36% of 50

B. 73.5% of 425

C. 25% of 350

D. 10% of 650

E. 12.5% of 700

CHANGING DECIMALS TO PERCENTS

Moving Decimals

The easy task of moving the decimal point is reversed to change decimals to percents. To rewrite a decimal to a percent, move the decimal point two (2) places to the right. For example, to write .75 as a percent:

$$75 = 75\%$$

To write .429 as a percent:

$$.429 = 42.9\%$$

Multiplying by 100

Since dividing by 100 converts a percent to a decimal, the opposite is done to convert a decimal to a percent. Moving the decimal point two places to the right is also the same as multiplying the number by 100. For example, to change .75 to a percent:

$$.75 \times 100 = 75\%$$

To change .429 to a percent:

$$.429 \times 100 = 42.9\%$$

Exercise 3

Convert these decimals to percentages. Try using both methods.

A. 0.10

B. 0.875

C. 0.06

D. 0.80

E. 0.167

Calculating Percentages

Another example is calculating the percentage grade on a test. If the student has 66 correct answers on a 75-question test, what is the student's percentage grade? The student's score is divided by the total possible points to arrive at the percentage grade the student will receive for the test.

$$66 \div 75 = 88\%$$

Exercise 4

In this example, the numbers are still divided to find the percent although the numbers are not based on a total of 100. Practice finding these percentages. Round up to the nearest two-digit percentage. For example, 99.1 rounds to 99 percent; 99.5 rounds to 100.

A. 32 out of 35

B. 109 out of 125

C. 43 out of 60

D. 19 out of 25

E. 385 out of 600

USING PERCENTAGES IN BILLING

Most insurance plans base the amount of reimbursement on a percentage of the amount billed. For example, an insurance plan uses an 80-20 policy (or 80-20 coinsurance), meaning that the insurance plan will reimburse 80 percent of the charges and the patient (or perhaps a supplemental insurance plan) is responsible for the remaining 20 percent of the charges.

Following that example, if the provider bills the patient $100 for an office visit, the insurance plan will reimburse the provider $80. The difference or remaining $20 is the responsibility of the patient to pay.

How did you arrive at these numbers? You need to calculate the percentages owed by each party.

$$
\begin{array}{rl}
\$100 & \text{Provider charges} \\
\times \quad 80\% & \text{Insurance plan reimbursement percentage} \\
\hline
\$80 & \text{Amount reimbursed by the insurance plan}
\end{array}
$$

$$
\begin{array}{rl}
\$100 & \text{Provider charges} \\
\times \quad 20\% & \text{Insurance plan non-reimbursement percentage} \\
\hline
\$20 & \text{Amount for which patient is responsible}
\end{array}
$$

Another method of completing the calculation is to determine the amount reimbursed by the insurance plan and then subtract to find the difference to be paid by the patient.

$$
\begin{array}{rl}
\$100 & \text{Provider charges} \\
\times \quad 80\% & \text{Insurance plan reimbursement percentage} \\
\hline
\$80 & \text{Amount reimbursed by the insurance plan}
\end{array}
$$

$$
\begin{array}{rl}
\$100 & \text{Provider charges} \\
- \quad \$80 & \text{Insurance plan reimbursement amount} \\
\hline
\$20 & \text{Amount for which patient is responsible}
\end{array}
$$

This information is then used by the medical insurance specialist, for example, in the patient's ledger card (also called the patient statement). On the day of the office visit, the charge of $100 is entered on the ledger card/patient statement. When the insurance claim is processed and reimbursed by the insurance plan, the payment received in the office is entered on the ledger card/patient statement and a new balance is calculated. Next, a statement or bill is sent to the patient. When the patient pays the amount owed, it is entered on the ledger card/patient statement and a new balance calculated, in this case a zero balance since the entire amount has been paid.

Example

Here is an example of a ledger card/patient statement for Harry Windsor, a patient with indemnity insurance. You can see that he was seen in the office on 7/2 and the charge was $100. The medical insurance specialist then submitted a health insurance claim to the insurance plan, which reimbursed the provider $80 on 7/13. A statement/bill was sent to the patient on 7/25, which is also noted on the ledger card/patient statement. A payment of $20 was received on 7/30, which reduced Mr. Windsor's balance to zero.

Harry Windsor 123 Buckingham Street Englishtown, NJ 07726		Pt. #214365 609-555-0764		Primary ins. - Northeast Secondary ins. - none	
Date/Pro		**Charge**	**Payment/Adj**		**Balance**
7/2	OV	100.00			100.00
7/3	INS	---		---	100.00
7/13	PMT		Insurance	80.00	20.00
7/25	STM	---		---	20.00
7/30	PMT		Patient	20.00	0.00

Exercise 5

Of course, not all percentages are calculated based on a $100 charge. Calculate the charges for the following patients.

A. Haiquao Wei is insured by an indemnity insurance plan that reimburses on a 75-25 basis. Mrs. Wei is seen in the office for a physical exam; the charges total $340. What is the amount to be billed to the insurance plan? What amount, if any, is due from the patient?

B. Irina Dombrowski's office exam had charges totaling $65. Her primary insurance is an indemnity plan with 85-15 coinsurance. What amount will be covered by the insurance plan? What amount, if any, will be billed to the patient?

In some instances, patients have insurance plans that include deductibles—amounts the patient must pay before insurance will begin to pay. When calculating charges for these patients, the medical insurance specialist must first calculate whether or not the patient has met the deductible. If so, the additional fees are reimbursed according to the insurance company's basis, such as 80-20.

Example

Justin Malozzi is insured by an HMO. For office visits within the network, he pays a copayment of $20. For out-of-network services there is a $150 deductible, then the plan reimburses on a 75-25 basis. Mr. Malozzi sought medical services from an out-of-network provider. For an office visit on 10/7, he had charges of $75. At his next office visit on 10/11, charges for a minor procedure totaled $123. Since Mr. Malozzi had not yet met his deductible, the medical insurance specialist calculated that he owed $150, and the remaining $48 would be submitted for reimbursement from PennCare Insurance. Under the policy, PennCare would pay 75 percent or $36 of the $48; Mr. Malozzi would be responsible for the remaining 25 percent or $12.

Justin Malozzi 4525 Maple Street Allentown, PA 18104		Pt. #852074 610-555-1597		Primary ins. – PennCare Secondary ins. - none
Date/Pro		**Charge**	**Payment/Adj**	**Balance**
10/7	OV	75.00		75.00
10/11	OV	123.00		198.00
10/11	PMT		Patient 150.00	48.00
11/1	PMT		PennCare 36.00	12.00
11/7	PMT		Patient 12.00	0.00

Exercise 6

Calculate the charges for these patients.

A. Jack Johnson has a high-deductible insurance policy. His deductible is $1,000 and reimbursement is on a 90-10 basis. To date, his charges have totaled $1,689. What amount is due from the insurance company? What amount is due from the patient?

B. Juanita Berrios has managed care insurance with a $20 copay for in-network providers. Use of an out-of-network provider means Juanita will have a $100 deductible and a 55-45 reimbursement. Juanita visited her in-network PCP on 4/13; the charge was $135. What amount is due from the patient?

C. Juanita (see the previous question) saw an out-of-network provider on 5/5; the charge was $212. What amount is due from the patient? What amount is reimbursed by the insurance company? Enter the information on her ledger card/patient statement. (There may be extra rows.)

Juanita Berrios	Pt. #483680	Primary ins. – Mgd. Care
721 Tamarack Street	610-555-3842	Secondary ins. - none
Allentown, PA 18105		

Date/Pro		Charge	Payment/Adj	Balance
4/13	OV	135.00		

APPLYING CONCEPTS

1. The patient's health insurance plan has a $750 deductible for hospital visits, and then covers 100 percent of hospital visit charges. The patient's first hospital visit this year had charges of $612. The patient was subsequently admitted to the hospital a second time this year and the charges totaled $358. How much will the patient be billed for each visit? How much will the health insurance plan reimburse for each visit?

2. A patient insured under an indemnity plan has an annual deductible for office visits of $100, after which the office plan covers 100 percent of fees, and requires a separate annual deductible for hospital coverage of $1,000, after which it covers 100 percent of charges. The patient was seen in the office, a normal office visit charge is $45, and was immediately sent to the hospital for an emergency appendectomy. The surgery charges totaled $7,382. How much, if anything, does the patient owe? To whom?

3. A patient in a POS plan has a $10 copayment and a 70-30 coinsurance rate on the balance of the charge. The patient is seen for an office visit; the total charge for the office visit is $85. What amount is owed by the patient?

4. Holly Hiker is insured by a HMO whose network is exclusive to her home city in Pennsylvania. The HMO expects patients to pay any costs up front when accessing health care services out of network; the patient then submits the

charges for 80 percent reimbursement except in emergency cases when 100 percent is reimbursed. She had a life-threatening injury while on a hiking vacation in Maine. She received treatment at the local trauma center's emergency room that totaled $1,732. What amount must Holly pay to the hospital in Maine? What amount will Holly be reimbursed by her HMO?

5. The patient has two insurance policies. Each policy's coinsurance is 80-20. If the patient has charges totaling $845, what amount should the medical insurance specialist expect to be reimbursed from Insurer A? From Insurer B? For what amount should the patient be billed?

6. The patient's insurance plan pays 80 percent of eye examinations for preventive care but does not pay for ophthalmology services related to refractions; the patient is responsible for these charges. The patient is examined by an ophthalmologist and prescribed corrective lenses. The bill is detailed as follows:

```
Ibrahim Ateyh
5/25/2016

Charges:
Complete eye exam      $95
Glaucoma check         N/C
Refraction exam        $65
Total                  $160
```

What amount is covered by the patient's insurance plan? What amount must the patient pay?

7. Sheena's health plan has a $250 deductible for each person or a maximum deductible of $1,000 for a family of more than four people per year. Once the deductible has been met, the plan reimburses on a 90-10 basis. Sheena's son, Shane, frequently sees a health care provider for a chronic illness. In fact, he was seen in the office on 1/16, 2/5, 2/26, 3/9, and 3/13 this year; his office visit charges total $375. Sheena's daughter, Sharon, had office visits on 1/20, 2/19, and a minor surgical procedure performed in the doctor's office on 2/20; her charges total $975. Sheena has now received a bill for her children's services through 3/31. What is the total amount due from the health plan? What is the total amount to be paid by Sheena?

For the following two calculations, refer to the insurance card shown in Case 1.1 on page 33 in Chapter 1.

8. Anthony is seen in your Connecticut office for an office visit and lab tests. He has not met his deductible for the year. The charges total $265. What amount is owed by the insurance plan? What amount is owed by the patient?

9. Anthony was seen in a physician's office and had lab tests in Utah, which is out of network. He has not met his deductible for the year. The total charges are $265. What amount is owed by the insurance plan? What amount is owed by the patient?

Chapter 2

Electronic Health Records, HIPAA, and HITECH: Sharing and Protecting Patients' Health Information

Learning Outcomes

After studying this chapter, you should be able to:

2.1 Explain the importance of accurate documentation when working with medical records.

2.2 Compare the intent of HIPAA and ARRA/HITECH laws.

2.3 Describe the relationship between covered entities and business associates.

2.4 Explain the purpose of the HIPAA Privacy Rule.

2.5 Briefly state the purpose of the HIPAA Security Rule.

2.6 Explain the purpose of the HITECH Breach Notification Rule.

2.7 Explain how the HIPAA Electronic Health Care Transactions and Code Sets standards influence the electronic exchange of health information.

2.8 Explain how to guard against potentially fraudulent situations.

2.9 Explain how various organizations enforce HIPAA.

2.10 Assess the benefits of a compliance plan.

ASSISTED OUTLINING

Directions: Read the chapter through one time. Then go back over the chapter and find the information required to complete the following outline of the chapter. Write the requested information directly in the spaces provided.

A medical insurance specialist reviews patients' medical records to:

   1.

   2.

3. A medical record must document what four things about services performed?

(1)   (3)

(2)   (4)

4. When and under what conditions may a medical insurance specialist legally share patient information?

2.1 Medical Record Documentation: Electronic Health Records

Medical Records

1. A patient's medical record provides _____ and _____ among _____ and _____ involved in a patient's care.

2. The concept of documentation means organizing a patient's health record in _____ order using a method that is _____, _____, and _____.

3. Explain the term *medical professional liability.*

4. What is the term to describe failure to meet medical standards of care resulting in injury or harm to the patient?

5. What is the basis for medical necessity?

Advantages of Electronic Health Records

6. Define electronic health records (EHR).

7. List eight advantages of EHRs over paper records.

(1)   (5)

(2)   (6)

(3)   (7)

(4)   (8)

8. There are three names/abbreviations used to describe types of computerized medical records. Name all three.

(1)   (3)

(2)

Documenting Encounters with Providers

List the information to be documented in every patient encounter:

9.

10.

11.

12.

13.

14.

15.

16.

17. List the nine Medicare standards for general documentation.

(1)   (6)

(2)   (7)

(3)   (8)

(4)   (9)

(5)

Evaluation and Management Services Reports

18. Define evaluation and management (E/M).

19. List the four types of information in a complete history and physical (H&P):

(1)   (3)

(2)   (4)

The history and physical examination section may also include:

(5)   (7)

(6)   (8)

20. How is informed consent usually obtained?

21. Patient progress notes include:

(1)   (3)

(2)   (4)

22. Discharge summaries include:

(1)   (4)

(2)   (5)

(3)   (6)

23. A procedure report is used to document:

(1)   (3)

(2)   (4)

Using PM/EHRs: An Integrated Medical Documentation and Billing Cycle

24. What explains how using EHRs is integrated with PMPs as the 10-step billing process is performed?

25. The reason for which a patient needs to see a doctor is known as what?

2.2 Health Care Regulation: HIPAA and HITECH

Federal Regulations

1. The main federal government agency responsible for health care is:

2. This agency was previously known as:

3. This agency is part of what federal department?

4. Another aspect of CMS is ensuring the quality of health care, such as

(1)   (3)

(2)   (4)

HIPAA

5. The most important recent legislation regulating health care is called the Health Insurance Portability and Accountability Act (HIPAA) of 1996. This law is designed to accomplish three goals:

(1)   (3)

(2)

HITECH

6. What is the purpose of the HITECH Act?

7. What is the title of the state officials who regulate the health care industry in each state?

8. What is meaningful use?

9. Into how many stages are incentives for achieving meaningful use divided?

10. What enables the sharing of health-related information among provider organizations according to nationally recognized standards?

ACA and Accountable Care Organizations

11. An accountable care organization (ACO) is a network of _____ and _____ that shares responsibility for managing the quality and cost of care provided to a group of patients.

2.3 Covered Entities and Business Associates

1. Patients' medical records—the actual progress notes, reports, and other materials—are legal documents that belong to:

2. The information contained in the patient's medical record belongs to:

3. Answers to questions such as what information in a patient's medical records can legally be shared with other providers are based on:

4. A key reason for HIPAA Administrative Simplification is Congress's wish to control costs by:

Electronic Data Interchange

5. Define electronic data interchange (EDI).

6. List the three parts to HIPAA's Administrative Simplification provisions:

(1)   (3)

(2)

Complying with HIPAA and HITECH

7. Define covered entities.

8. List the three types of covered entities that must follow the regulations:

(1)   (3)

(2)

9. What practices are not considered a covered entity?

10. Define business associates in relation to covered entities.

2.4 HIPAA Privacy Rule

1. What is the HIPAA Privacy Rule and what does it protect?

2. The HIPAA Privacy Rule says that covered entities must

(1)   (4)

(2)   (5)

(3)

Protected Health Information

3. Define protected health information (PHI).

4. What type of information is included in PHI?

(1)	(9)
(2)	(10)
(3)	(11)
(4)	(12)
(5)	(13)
(6)	(14)
(7)	(15)
(8)	(16)

Use and Disclosure for Treatment, Payment, and Health Care Operations

5. Explain the difference between use of PHI and disclosure of PHI.

6. No patient release of information document is needed when PHI is shared for:

Examples of HIPAA Compliance

7. What is not included in the designated record set (DRS) for a provider?

8. What is included in the designated record set (DRS) for a health plan?

9. Within the designated record set, patients have the right to

(1)	(4)
(2)	(5)
(3)	

10. When should patients receive their Notice of Privacy Practices (NPP)?

Authorizations for Other Use and Disclosure

11. The authorization to release information document is signed by the patient and must be in plain language and must include the following:

(1)	(6)
(2)	(7)
(3)	(8)
(4)	(9)
(5)	

Exceptions

12. List five situations in which there could be exceptions to the usual rules for release of information other than TPO.

(1)   (4)

(2)   (5)

(3)

De-identified Health Information

13. What is de-identified health information?

Psychotherapy Notes

14. What items from psychotherapy notes are not included in the patient's chart under psychotherapy notes?

State Statutes

15. If a state statute is more stringent than a HIPAA rule, which is followed?

2.5 HIPAA Security Rule

1. Explain the HIPAA Security Rule.

Encryption Is Required

2. What is the process of encoding information in such a way that only the person (or computer) with the key can decode it?

Security Measures

3. List three other security measures that help enforce the HIPAA Security Rule.

(1)   (3)

(2)

2.6 HITECH Breach Notification Rule

1. Define breach as it relates to the HITECH Act.

Breach Notification Procedures

2. What must a covered entity do when a breach occurs?

3. What is the document notifying an individual of a breach called?

4. Name the five points that must be included in a breach notification.

(1)   (4)

(2)   (5)

(3)

2.7 HIPAA Electronic Health Care Transactions and Code Sets

1. The HIPAA Electronic Health Care Transactions and Code Sets (TCS) standards have both a _____ beginning with an X and a _____.

Standard Transactions

2. List the seven standards (TCS) using both the number and name.

Number	Official Name
(1)	
(2)	
(3)	
(4)	
(5)	
(6)	
(7)	

Standard Code Sets

3. List four code sets used for encoding data elements:

(1)   (3)

(2)   (4)

HIPAA National Identifiers

4. List the two existing HIPAA National Identifiers:

(1)   (2)

5. What did the NPI replace?

2.8 Fraud and Abuse Regulations

The Health Care Fraud and Abuse Control Program

1. The Health Care Fraud and Abuse Control Program that uncovers and prosecutes fraud and abuse is enforced by three different agencies. List each agency and the types of violations they enforce.

(1)   (3)

(2)

False Claims Act, Fraud Enforcement and Recovery Act, and State Laws

2. Under the federal False Claims Act (FCA), what is prohibited?

3. Define *qui tam*.

Additional Laws

4. List three additional laws relating to health care fraud and abuse control.

(1)   (3)

(2)

Definition of Fraud and Abuse

5. Explain the difference between fraud and abuse.

2.9 Enforcement and Penalties

1. When was the HIPAA final enforcement rule implemented?

Office of Inspector General

2. What is the purpose of an OIG audit?

2.10 Compliance Plans

1. Define *respondeat superior*.

2. A compliance plan sets up the steps needed to:

(1)   (3)

(2)   (4)

3. List the goals of a HIPAA compliance plan:

(1)   (3)

(2)

Parts of a Compliance Plan

4. List the seven OIG approved elements usually contained in a voluntary compliance plan.

(1)   (5)

(2)   (6)

(3)   (7)

(4)

Compliance Officer and Committee

5. Who is the person responsible for establishing the plan and following-up on its provisions?

Code of Conduct

6. List three elements of the code of conduct for practice members.

(1)   (3)

(2)

Ongoing Training

7. An important part of the compliance plan is a commitment to
_____.

KEY TERMS

Defining

Define each of the following terms.

Abuse	HIPAA Security Rule
Audit	Malpractice
Breach	Medical records
Compliance plan	Medical standards of care
Covered entity	National Provider Identifier
De-identified health information	Protected health information
Fraud	TPO
HIPAA Privacy Rule	

SELF-QUIZ

1. When sending information electronically using a computer, how can you tell if it is protected?

2. Give an example of a poor password choice.

3. Who owns the information contained in the medical record? The paper medical record?

4. If a patient's PHI is included in a health care claim transmission, is authorization needed from the patient? Why or why not?

CRITICAL THINKING QUESTIONS

1. As a consumer of health care services, what advantages and disadvantages are there to electronic health records?

2. Is there a difference between fraud and abuse?

3. Should spouses have the right to view each other's medical record without authorization?

4. What is the benefit of having business associates adhere to the provisions of HIPAA?

5. List some guidelines for creating effective passwords.

WEB ACTIVITIES

SURFING THE NET

1. View the .pdf file of the entire HIPAA act at:
   www.cms.gov/HIPAAGenInfo/Downloads/HIPAAlawdetail.pdf. In section
   1176, General Penalty, what are the penalties that can be imposed for HIPAA
   violations?

   _____

   _____

2. In 2004, the President's Information Technology Advisory Committee made
   recommendations regarding medical records and information technology. In a
   letter to President Bush on June 30, 2004, they suggested four core elements
   as a basis for improving medical records systems. The report can be found at
   www.nitrd.gov/pitac/reports/20040721_hit_report.pdf. The four core
   elements of this framework are:

   (1) _____   (3) _____

   (2) _____   (4) _____

USING THE WEB WISELY

1. Using more than one search engine such as Google or Yahoo, enter the term
   Electronic Health Records Software.

   A. How many possible hits did you find in each search?

   _____

   B. Evaluate a few of the hits to understand what is provided in that
      program's/company's electronic solutions for medical records.

   _____

2. Go to the website for Medisoft, www.medisoft.com/.

   A. How does Medisoft compare to the results from question 1B?

   _____

APPLYING CONCEPTS

1. An employee of Riverside Family Practice is having difficulty getting all the faxed lab reports placed into patient files each week. She decides to take the charts and faxed lab reports home over the weekend to get caught up on the filing. What are the legal implications for the employee and the practice due to this action? What are the ethical implications?

2. You receive a telephone call from a person who says she is one of your practice's patients, Leslie Van Arsdale, requesting the results of her lab tests. How can you verify that the person is, in fact, Ms. Van Arsdale?

3. You have the opportunity to design the patient privacy authorization form(s). What are the steps in planning the form(s)? What specific types of release of information need to be covered?

4. Read the following entry in the medical record of Charlie Chevalier. What is missing from this record? The transcriptionist, Juanita Brazos, noticed an error immediately after printing. She then noted a correction. Is the correction done properly? Are there any other errors in transcription?

CHART NOTE

Charlie
October 2016

CC: Acne of face and back

Vital signs: B/P 118/86 Pulse 78 Weight 147

I last saw this 22-year-old white male 2 months ago for an initial office visit due to complaints of acne on his face and upper back. At that time I placed him on ampicillin and Neutrogena Acne Wash. At this time he shows little to no improvement, actually showing more comedo formation and more pustular lesions than before. The lesions are now more prominent over his entire upper back. He is on no other medications and is otherwise in good health.

The patient has both blackheads and whiteheads over the chin, along the jaw line, on the skin of the neck, and over the forehead. Approximately 525% of the lesions on the face are inflamed show inflammatory reaction, and approximately 10% of the lesions on the upper back are inflamed.

four times JB 10/12/2016

Medications will be changed to Benzamycin 2% gel to be used topically ~~twice~~ daily after washing and Vibramycin 250mg b.i.d. orally. He has been reminded to avoid touching his face as much as possible and to not pick the lesions. He will be seen again in 4 to 6 weeks.

Li Wu, MD

LW/jb
D: 10/12/2016
T: 10/12/2016

Chapter 3 Patient Encounters and Billing Information

Learning Outcomes

After studying this chapter, you should be able to:

3.1 Explain the method used to classify patients as new or established.

3.2 Discuss the five categories of information required of new patients.

3.3 Explain how information for established patients is updated.

3.4 Verify patients' eligibility for insurance benefits.

3.5 Discuss the importance of requesting referral or preauthorization approval.

3.6 Determine primary insurance for patients who have more than one health plan.

3.7 Summarize the use of encounter forms.

3.8 Identify the eight types of charges that may be collected from patients at the time of service.

3.9 Explain the use of real-time claims adjudication tools in calculating time-of-service payments.

ASSISTED OUTLINING

Directions: Read the chapter through one time. Then go back over the chapter and find the information required to complete the following outline of the chapter. Write the requested information directly in the spaces provided.

1. List the three parts of processing patient encounters for billing purposes:

   (1)   (3)

   (2)

3.1 New Versus Established Patients

1. Explain the difference between a new patient and an established patient.

3.2 Information for New Patients

1. List the five types of information most important about a new patient:

   (1)   (4)

   (2)   (5)

   (3)

Preregistration and Scheduling Information

2. What basic information is gathered from a new or an established patient when scheduling an appointment?

   (1)   (5)

   (2)   (6)

   (3)   (7)

   (4)   (8)

Preregistration and Scheduling Information

3. Define PAR.

Medical History

4. What types of information are collected on the new patient medical history form (an example is shown in Figure 3.2 in your textbook)? What is done with this information?

Patient/Guarantor and Insurance Data

5. A typical patient information form (also called a patient registration form) collects many items of demographic data about the patient. What are they? (An example is shown in Figure 3.3 in your textbook.)

   (1)   (9)

   (2)   (10)

   (3)   (11)

   (4)   (12)

   (5)   (13)

   (6)   (14)

   (7)   (15)

   (8)   (16)

Insurance Cards

6. What are six of the typical types of information found on insurance cards?

(1)   (4)

(2)   (5)

(3)   (6)

Photo Identification

7. If a photo ID is presented, what procedure is followed?

Assignment of Benefits

8. Explain assignment of benefits.

Acknowledgment of Receipt of Notice of Privacy Practices

9. What does TPO stand for?

10. Under HIPAA, define the types of information covered for TPO (define each letter separately).

(1)   (3)

(2)

11. What are the typical procedures involved in informing patients about the provider's privacy practices?

3.3 Information for Established Patients

1. How can the medical insurance specialist assure timely and correct information about established patients?

Entering Patient Information in the Practice Management Program

2. A practice management program uses two main databases of information. They are:

(1)   (2)

Communications with Patients

3. Medical insurance specialists often handle patients' questions about benefits and charges. They must become:

3.4 Verifying Patient Eligibility for Insurance Benefits

1. List the steps to establish financial responsibility.

   (1)   (3)

   (2)

2. What three points are verified by contacting the payer?

   (1)   (3)

   (2)

Factors Affecting General Eligibility

3. What are some of the factors that affect eligibility for insurance benefits?

4. What is the HIPAA Standard Transaction number to electronically send an inquiry or receive a response regarding eligibility for a health plan?

Checking Out-Of-Network Benefits

5. If a patient has insurance coverage with no out-of-network benefits, and the practice does not participate in the patient's plan, what portion of the bill is the patient responsible for?

Verifying the Amount of the Copayment or Coinsurance

6. Why should the amount of the copayment be verified?

Determining Whether the Planned Encounter Is for a Covered Service

7. Why is it important to determine in advance if the planned service(s) are covered service(s)?

Electronic Benefit Inquiries and Responses

8. More than ten pieces of information are used to respond to an eligibility inquiry. List at least six.

   (1)   (4)

   (2)   (5)

   (3)   (6)

Procedures When the Patient Is Not Covered

9. Who is responsible for payment if an insured patient's policy does not cover a planned service?

3.5 Determining Preauthorization and Referral Requirements

Preauthorization

1. How is preauthorization requested from a health plan?

2. What is the HIPAA Standard Transaction number to electronically send an inquiry for preauthorization or certification from a health plan?

Referrals

3. When a patient is referred to another provider, what must the office handling the referred patient do?

(1)   (3)

(2)

3.6 Determining the Primary Insurance

1. Explain the difference between primary and secondary insurance.

2. Is it possible for patients to have more than two insurance plans? If so, what terms are used to refer to these additional insurance plans?

3. Explain coordination of benefits.

4. What is the HIPAA Standard Transaction number to electronically send an inquiry for coordination of benefits?

Guidelines for Determining the Primary Insurance

5. List the guidelines for determining which insurance is the primary insurance when a patient has two or more health plans:

(1)   (7)

(2)   (a)

(3)   (b)

(4)   (c)

(5)   (8)

(6)   (9)

Guidelines for Children with More than One Insurance Plan

6. Explain the birthday rule and its application to children whose parents both have an insurance plan that covers dependent children.

7. How is insurance coverage determined for children whose parents are separated or divorced and have joint custody?

8. If parents do not have joint custody of the child (and a court order is not in effect), how is the primary insurance determined?

    (1)   (3)

    (2)

Entering Insurance Information in the Practice Management Program

9. The medical insurance specialist updates the practice management program as needed to reflect the patient's primary _____ _____.

Communications with Payers

10. List three guidelines for effective communications with payers:

    (1)   (3)

    (2)

3.7 Working with Encounter Forms

1. What information is usually preprinted on the encounter form?

2. What information does the provider place on the encounter form?

3. What are alternate names for the encounter form?

Paper Preprinted or Computer-Generated Encounter Forms

4. What is the purpose of numbering encounter forms?

3.8 Understanding Time-of-Service (TOS) Payments

Routine Collections at the Time of Service

1. What payments are routinely collected at the time of service?

    (1)   (5)

    (2)   (6)

    (3)   (7)

    (4)   (8)

Copayments

2. Can the copayment vary by type of service?

Coinsurance

3. Why is coinsurance becoming more common?

Charges for Noncovered/Overlimit Services

4. Who is responsible for payment for services not covered by the health plan or services provided once all benefits have been used?

Charges of Nonparticipating Providers

5. Give an explanation of accepting assignment.

6. What is the difference between PAR and nonPAR?

Charges for Services to Self-pay Patients

7. Who are self-pay patients?

Other TOS Collection Considerations

8. To increase time-of-service collections, how may practices change their billing process?

3.9 Calculating TOS Payments

Financial Policy and Health Plan Provisions

1. What is a financial policy? How is it communicated to patients?

Estimating What the Patient Will Owe

2. What steps are taken to estimate charges?

Real-time Claims Adjudication

3. Explain the three steps in RTCA (real-time claims adjudication).

(1)   **(3)**

(2)

Financial Arrangements for Large Bills

4. A financial arrangement involves a _____ of payments.

KEY TERMS

Multiple Choice

Circle the letter of the choice that best matches the definition or answers the question.

1. To file claims for the patient and receive payments directly from the payer to the provider.

   A. Prior authorization number
   B. Participating provider
   C. Partial payment
   D. Accept assignment

2. This patient has seen the provider (or another provider in the practice who has the same specialty) within the past three years.

   A. Established patient
   B. Referred patient
   C. New patient
   D. Surgical patient

3. These guidelines ensure that when a patient has more than one policy, maximum appropriate benefits are paid, but without duplication.

   A. Walkout receipt
   B. HIPAA Security Rule
   C. Coordination of benefits
   D. Prior authorization number

4. This person is the holder of the insurance policy that covers the patient, and is not necessarily also a patient of the practice.

   A. Referring physician
   B. Specialist
   C. Purchaser
   D. Insured

5. Patients who do not have insurance coverage are called:

   A. New patients
   B. Self-pay patients
   C. Established patients
   D. Returning patients

6. The health insurance plan that pays first when more than one plan is in effect.

   A. Supplemental insurance
   B. Tertiary insurance
   C. Secondary insurance
   D. Primary insurance

7. This form includes a patient's personal, employment, and insurance company data.

   A. Encounter form
   B. Authorization form
   C. Claim form
   D. Patient information form

8. A provider that does not accept assignment from a particular health plan.

   A. Referring physician
   B. Participating provider
   C. Nonparticipating provider
   D. PCP

9. The process used to determine the primary insurance if both parents cover dependents on their health insurance plans.

   A. Gender rule
   B. HIPAA Privacy Rule
   C. Birthday rule
   D. Referral waiver

10. A form used to collect basic demographic information about the patient.

   A. Encounter form
   B. Patient information form
   C. Coordination of benefits
   D. Authorization form

CRITICAL THINKING QUESTIONS

1. Should the gender rule be used to determine primary insurance for dependent children? Why or why not?

2. If the patient cannot (or will not) pay the copay or coinsurance at the time of the office visit, should services be withheld except in cases of emergency?

3. How does asking for the chief complaint or reason for the office visit at the time of scheduling help you effectively plan?

4. Who is ultimately responsible for payment of charges incurred for medical services?

5. What are three types of information captured on the Patient Information Form? How is each type used?

WEB ACTIVITIES

SURFING THE NET

1. Using a search engine such as Google or Yahoo, locate the website of the CHIP program in your state.

   (a) What types of services are covered under CHIP?

   _____

   _____

   (b) What are the eligibility requirements for children?

   _____

   _____

   (c) What are the income guidelines for families to be eligible for CHIP?

   _____

   _____

   (d) What is the monthly cost for coverage?

   _____

   _____

   (e) How many different health plans are offered?

   _____

   _____

2. Using your favorite browser, go to www.healthcare-informatics.com/index.php (or use a search engine to locate the article) and search for information on HIPAA and security.

   (a) Locate a recent article that specifically gives suggestions or tips for physician offices on an issue related to HIPAA and security.

   _____

   _____

   (b) Summarize the information to share with your instructor. Remember to include a reference citation.

   _____

   _____

WEB SCAVENGER HUNT

3. Using a search engine such as Google or Yahoo, locate information on RHIOs.

   (a) What is an RHIO?
   (b) What are some of the advantages of participating in an RHIO?
   (c) What are some of the disadvantages of participating in an RHIO?
   (d) Is there an RHIO in your area? Does your local hospital participate?

USING MATH IN THE MEDICAL OFFICE

For review, refer to the first chapter on how to calculate percentages.

USING PERCENTAGES IN BILLING

Many patients have more than one insurance plan. For the medical billing specialist this means that claims may be sent to more than one insurance plan. Previously only examples wherein the patient had one insurance plan were used. Now try calculating the billing when a patient has two insurance plans.

   The medical insurance specialist first determines which plan is the primary insurance—the plan that pays first—and checks to see what deductibles, copayments, coinsurance, etc., are applied to the charges. The billing is calculated and entered on the ledger card/patient statement. Then a claim is sent to the primary insurance plan. When payment(s) is received, the medical insurance specialist enters the payments on the ledger card/patient statement.

   Next, the medical insurance specialist identifies the secondary insurance plan and follows the same steps, completing the necessary calculations and entering the data on the patient's ledger card/patient statement. A claim is created and sent to the secondary insurance plan. Any payment(s) received are entered on the ledger card/patient statement.

   In the final step, the medical insurance specialist calculates any charges not reimbursed by the insurance plans and bills the patient. When payment is received, it is entered on the ledger card/patient statement.

   Let's use an example of a $100 charge.

$100	Provider charges
× 80%	Insurance plan 1 reimbursement percentage
$80	Amount reimbursed by insurance plan 1
$20	Charges not reimbursed by insurance plan 1
× 80%	Insurance plan 2 reimbursement percentage
$16	Amount reimbursed by insurance plan 2
$20	Charges not reimbursed by insurance plan 1
− $16	Charges reimbursed by insurance plan 2
$ 4	Amount for which patient is responsible

The concept of coordination of benefits (COB) is also illustrated here, since each insurer pays only that portion for which it is responsible, but the total reimbursement does not exceed the total amount of the charges.

Example

Here is an example of a ledger card/patient statement for Linda Ragou, a patient with indemnity insurance that has a coinsurance of 80-20. Her spouse, Franco, also has indemnity insurance with a coinsurance of 80-20. She was seen in the office on 9/22 and the charge was $100. The medical insurance specialist then submitted a health insurance claim to the primary insurance plan, which reimbursed the provider $80 (80% × $100) on 9/29. This payment was entered in Mrs. Ragou's ledger card/patient statement on the same date. On 9/30 the medical insurance specialist submitted a health insurance claim to the secondary insurance plan, which reimbursed the provider $16 (80% × $20). This payment was entered on 10/3, the same day it was received. A statement/bill was sent to the patient on 10/5, which is also noted on the ledger card/patient statement. A payment of $4 was received on 10/13, which reduced Ms. Ragou's balance to zero.

Linda Ragou 312 Adams Avenue Bethlehem, PA 18020		Pt. #663921 610-555-5881		Primary ins. – Midwest(pt.) Secondary ins. – Central(spouse) Spouse – Franco Ragou	
Date/Pro		**Charge**	**Payment/Adj**		**Balance**
9/22	OV	100.00			100.00
9/23	INS1	---		---	100.00
9/29	PMT		INS1	80.00	20.00
9/30	INS2	---		---	20.00
10/3	PMT		INS2	16.00	4.00
10/5	STM	---		---	4.00
10/13	PMT		Patient	4.00	0.00

APPLYING CONCEPTS

1. The patient is insured by a PPO with 100 percent coverage after a copay of $15. The patient was seen in the office for a checkup, and the total charges were $115. What amount must the patient pay? When? What amount must the insurance plan pay? When?

2. Afaf Darcy is insured by an HMO with a $10 copay and out-of-network coinsurance on charge balances of 90-10. She needed physical therapy after her knee replacement. Her HMO pays for 18 physical therapy sessions in such cases at a rate of $63.50 per visit. If additional physical therapy is needed, the provider must document the reasons and submit a formal request. The therapist requested additional visits, and Ms. Darcy attended 5 additional physical therapy sessions. The request was denied. What amount will the insurance company pay for her physical therapy? What amount must Ms. Darcy pay?

3. Mike Moroni is covered by a member health plan with a 20 percent discount from the provider's usual fees and a $20.00 copay. The charges are $365.50. What amount will the HMO pay? What does the patient owe?

4. Lisa Perez was seen in your office twice last fall. Her deductible has been met and her coinsurance is 85-15. In October, she was seen for influenza vaccination and her insurance company was billed $13.00 for the vaccine and $9.00 for the administration of the vaccine. Lisa's schedule of benefits for her indemnity insurance plan lists the influenza administration as being a covered service, but it does not include the actual vaccine. In December, Lisa had an office visit and had blood drawn to be sent to an outside lab; both these services are included in the schedule of benefits.

The ledger card/patient statement shows the dates and charges for services; you need to calculate each amount paid by the insurance plan and enter it on the ledger card/patient statement. Remember to keep a running balance.

Lisa Perez 478 Third Street Allentown, PA 18102 610-555-1937				Universal Health Chart #753159	
Date	**Description**	**Provider**	**Charge**	**Payment**	**Balance**
10/13	Influenza virus vaccine	sek	13.00		
10/13	Administration influenza	sek	9.00		
10/25	Ins rej. serv. not covered				
10/25	Plan payment				
12/19	OV/outpt. Est 99213	ll	65.00		
12/19	Drawing blood fee	ll	5.00		
12/29	Plan payment OV				
12/29	Plan payment veinpuncture				

5. Harold and Helen Rubright's coverage is with a consumer driven PPO with a high deductible of $1,000. The patient must pay a $25 copay for office visits. Previously, Mr. Rubright was seen in the office for a minor surgical procedure with charges totaling $1,000. The PPO was billed to maintain a record of the deductible; Mr. Rubright paid $1,000 on 5/5. These entries are shown on the ledger card/patient statement.

On 6/23 Mrs. Rubright was seen for an office visit. Charges were $65. Make the next two entries on the ledger card/patient statement.

Mr. Rubright was seen for an office visit on 10/7. Charges were $115. Make the necessary entries in the ledger card/patient statement.

Harold Rubright		MetropolisCare	
67 Blue Barn Road		Chart #852753	
Allentown, PA 18105			
610-555-1048			
Date/Pro	Charge	Payment/Adj	Balance
4/13 Surgery	1,000.00		1,000.00
4/23 INS	---	---	1,000.00
5/5 PMT		Patient 1,000.00	0.0
6/23 OV	65.00		65.00
6/23 Copay			
6/27 INS			
10/7			

Chapter 4 Diagnostic Coding: ICD-10-CM

Learning Outcomes

After studying this chapter, you should be able to:

4.1 Discuss the purpose of ICD-10-CM.

4.2 Describe the organization of ICD-10-CM.

4.3 Summarize the structure, content, and key conventions of the Alphabetic Index.

4.4 Summarize the structure, content, and key conventions of the Tabular List.

4.5 Apply the rules for outpatient coding that are provided in the ICD-10-CM *Official Guidelines for Coding and Reporting*.

4.6 Briefly describe the content of Chapters 1 through 21 of the Tabular List.

4.7 Assign correct ICD-10-CM diagnosis codes.

4.8 Differentiate between ICD-9-CM and ICD-10-CM.

ASSISTED OUTLINING

Directions: Read the chapter through one time. Then go back over the chapter and find the information required to complete the following outline of the chapter. Write the requested information directly in the spaces provided.

1. What is the purpose of a coding system?

2. Who may assign or determine a diagnosis?

3. Who may assign or determine a diagnosis code?

4.1 ICD-10-CM

1. What is the ICD-10?

2. Who developed the ICD-10?

3. What does ICD-10-CM stand for?

4. What is the difference between the ICD-10 and the ICD-10-CM?

5. How is the ICD-10-CM used?

Code Makeup

6. In what format are ICD-10-CM codes?

7. What lengths of ICD-10-CM codes are valid?

8. When sixth and seventh characters are available for assignment in the ICD-10-CM code set, must they be used?

Updates

9. What are updates to the ICD-10-CM called?

10. When must new ICD-10-CM codes be used?

4.2 Organization of ICD-10-CM

1. List and describe the two major parts of ICD-10-CM.

(1)   (2)

2. List and describe the three additional sections of the ICD-10-CM's first part that provide resources for researching correct codes.

(1)   (3)

(2)

3. The process of assigning ICD-10-CM codes begins with the physician's
   _____.

4. What are typographic techniques that provide visual guidance for understanding information in ICD-10-CM called?

4.3 The Alphabetic Index

1. How is the Alphabetic Index organized?

Main Terms, Subterms, and Nonessential Modifiers

2. Define main term as used in the Alphabetic Index. How are main terms displayed in the Alphabetic Index?

3. How are subterms used? How are they displayed in the Alphabetic Index?

4. How and where are nonessential modifiers shown?

Common Terms

   5. What is the common term for influenza?

Eponyms

   6. Define eponym. Give an example.

Indention: Turnover Lines

   7. What is a turnover line? How is it displayed in the Alphabetic Index?

Cross-References

   8. Explain the difference between *see* and *see also* in cross-references.

The Abbreviations NEC and NOS

   9. How is NEC used?

   10. How is NOS used?

Multiple Codes, Connecting Words, and Combination Codes

   11. What is a manifestation?

   12. What does the use of brackets around a code in the Alphabetic Index mean?

   13. What is a combination code?

4.4 The Tabular List

   1. How is the Tabular List organized?

   2. What are the 21 chapters used in the tabular list?

(1)	(12)
(2)	(13)
(3)	(14)
(4)	(15)
(5)	(16)
(6)	(17)
(7)	(18)
(8)	(19)
(9)	(20)
(10)	(21)
(11)	

3. How is a placeholder character designated?

4. Where is the seventh-character extension requirement contained?

Categories, Subcategories, and Codes

5. Explain category and subcategory.

(1)   **(2)**

6. The first character in a code is always _____.

Inclusion Notes

7. What are inclusion notes?

Exclusion Notes

8. What are exclusion notes?

9. What is the difference between the two types of exclusion notes?

Punctuation

10. Explain the meaning of the following:

(1) Colons :   **(3)** Brackets [ ]

(2) Parentheses ( )

Etiology/Manifestation Coding

11. A statement that a condition is _____ or _____ may require an additional code.

12. What does the instruction *use an additional code* mean?

13. What does the instruction *code first underlying disease* (or similar wording) mean?

Laterality

14. What is the concept of laterality as used in ICD-10-CM?

4.5 ICD-10-CM Official Guidelines for Coding and Reporting

1. What groups comprise the four cooperating parties that develop the *ICD-10-CM Official Guidelines for Coding and Reporting*?

   (1)   (3)

   (2)   (4)

2. What is one major reason to adhere to the *Official Guidelines*?

3. What are the three general rules for coding according to the *Official Guidelines*?

   (1)   (3)

   (2)

Code the Primary Diagnosis First, Followed by Current Coexisting Conditions

4. Explain the order used to list diagnosis codes.

Coding Acute versus Chronic Conditions

5. Explain the difference between acute and chronic conditions.

Coding Sequelae

6. Define sequelae.

Code the Highest Level of Certainty

7. Are inconclusive diagnoses used to determine the first-listed codes reported for reimbursement of service fees?

Signs and Symptoms

8. What is the difference between a *sign* and a *symptom*?

Suspected Conditions

9. What is the first-listed diagnosis referred to as in hospital coding?

Coding the Reason for Surgery

10. What diagnosis is used to code surgery?

Code to the Highest Level of Specificity

11. The more characters a code has, _____.

4.6 Overview of ICD-10-CM Chapters

A00–B99 Certain Infectious and Parasitic Diseases

1. In this chapter, most categories describe a _____ and the type of _____ that causes it.

C00–D49 Neoplasms

2. What is a neoplasm?

3. Name the six columns that relate to the behavior of a neoplasm.

(1)   (4)

(2)   (5)

(3)   (6)

4. What is the purpose of M codes?

D50–D89 Diseases of the Blood and Blood-forming Organs and Certain Disorders Involving the Immune Mechanism

5. Give an example of a condition that would fall in this chapter.

E00–E89 Endocrine, Nutritional, and Metabolic Diseases

6. What is the most common disease in this chapter?

F01–F99 Mental and Behavioral Disorders

7. This chapter includes codes for conditions of _____ and _____ dependency.

G00–G99 Diseases of the Nervous System

8. This chapter has codes for disease of the _____ nervous system and the _____ nervous system.

H00–H59 Diseases of the Eyes and Adnexa

9. This chapter contains codes for diseases of the _____ and _____.

H60–H95 Diseases of the Ear and Mastoid Process

10. This chapter contains codes for diseases of the _____ and _____.

I00–I99 Diseases of the Circulatory System

11. The notes and _____ instructions must be carefully observed to code circulatory diseases accurately.

J00–J99 Diseases of the Respiratory System

12. What does COPD stand for?

K00–K94 Diseases of the Digestive System

13. In this chapter, codes are listed according to anatomical location, beginning with the _____.

L00–L99 Diseases of the Skin and Subcutaneous Tissue

14. Codes in this chapter classify _____.

M00–M99 Diseases of the Musculoskeletal System and Connective Tissue

15. In this chapter, codes are provided for both _____ and _____.

N00–N99 Diseases of the Genitourinary System

16. Codes in this chapter classify diseases of both the _____ and _____ genitourinary systems.

O00–O9A Pregnancy, Childbirth, and the Puerperium

17. What is the puerperium?

P00–P96 Certain Conditions Originating in the Perinatal Period

18. What is a neonate?

Q00–Q99 Congenital Malformations, Deformations, and Chromosomal Abnormalities

19. What are congenital conditions?

R00–R99 Symptoms, Signs, and Abnormal Clinical and Laboratory Findings, Not Elsewhere Classified

20. Codes in this chapter classify patients' signs, symptoms, and ill-defined conditions for which a _____ cannot be made.

S00–T88 Injury, Poisoning, and Certain Other Consequences of External Causes

21. In addition to codes from this chapter, codes from _____ are often used to identify the cause of the injury or poisoning.

V00–Y99 External Causes of Morbidity

22. What are external cause codes?

23. How are external cause codes located?

24. What are Z codes?

25. Describe the two chief types of Z codes.

(1)   (2)

4.7 Coding Steps

1. List the six steps to correctly assign accurate diagnosis codes:

(1)   (4)

(2)   (5)

(3)   (6)

Step 1: Review Complete Medical Documentation

2. Explain the difference between the chief complaint and primary diagnosis.

Step 2: Abstract the Medical Conditions from the Visit Documentation

3. The code will be assigned based on the _____.

Step 3: Identify the Main Term for Each Condition

4. How can a condition be found?

Step 4: Locate the Main Term in the Alphabetic Index

5. What five guidelines should be followed when using the Alphabetic Index for selecting the correct term?

(1)   (4)

(2)   (5)

(3)

Step 5: Verify the Code in the Tabular List

6. What four guidelines should be followed when using the Tabular List for selecting the correct code?

(1)   (3)

(2)   (4)

Step 6: Check Compliance with Any Applicable Office Guidelines and List Codes in Appropriate Order

7. What should coders keep in mind when checking their code selection?

4.8 ICD-10-CM and ICD-9-CM

1. Name the two major advantages that ICD-10-CM provides over ICD-9-CM.

(1)   **(2)**

Differences and Similarities between ICD-9-CM and ICD-10-CM

2. Name some of the major differences between ICD-10-CM and ICD-9-CM.

(1)   **(4)**

(2)   **(5)**

(3)   **(6)**

3. Name the two major similarities that exist between the code sets.

(1)   **(2)**

GEMS

4. What does GEMs stand for?

5. What entity prepared GEMs?

KEY TERMS

MATCHING

Match the definition with the correct term from the following word list.

A. acute	F. NEC (not elsewhere classified)
B. late effect	G. eponym
C. chief complaint	H. NOS (not otherwise specified)
D. manifestation	I. etiology
E. chronic	J. primary diagnosis

(1) The cause or origin of a disease or condition.

(2) A residual condition that remains after a patient's acute illness or injury has ended.

(3) A disease's typical signs, symptoms, or secondary processes.

(4) An abbreviation indicating the code to use when a disease or condition cannot be placed in any other category.

(5) Conditions that continue over a long period of time or recur frequently.

(6) An abbreviation indicating the code to use when no information is available for assigning the disease or condition a more specific code.

(7) A patient's description of the symptoms or other reasons for seeking medical care.

(8) An illness or condition with severe symptoms and a short duration.

(9) A condition (or a procedure) named for a person.

(10) The first-listed diagnosis.

SELF-QUIZ

1. List the twenty-one chapters, and the corresponding code series, of the ICD-10-CM.

(1)	**(12)**
(2)	**(13)**
(3)	**(14)**
(4)	**(15)**
(5)	**(16)**
(6)	**(17)**
(7)	**(18)**
(8)	**(19)**
(9)	**(20)**
(10)	**(21)**
(11)	

2. If the Alphabetic Index has the words *see also* after an entry, what should the medical insurance specialist do?

3. Identify at least three eponyms.

(1)	**(3)**
(2)	

4. Explain how main terms and default codes appear in the Alphabetic Index.

5. How are entries listed in the Alphabetic Index?

6. For the following terms, underline the main terms once and underline the subterms twice:

   (1) Incomplete bundle branch heart block

   (2) Cerebral atherosclerosis

   (3) Acute bacterial food poisoning

   (4) Skin test for hypersensitivity

   (5) Spasmodic asthma with status asthmaticus

CRITICAL THINKING QUESTIONS

1. Why did the Medicare Catastrophic Coverage Act of 1988 require the use of codes rather than diagnostic statements?

2. Why is it important for WHO to standardize codes to be used worldwide?

3. Why can't the medical insurance specialist use a code book from a previous year?

4. The code numbers are listed in the Alphabetic Index. Why not code directly from it?

WEB ACTIVITIES

SURFING THE NET

Using a search engine such as Google or Yahoo, search for the ICD-10-CM.

1. How many vendors can you identify that sell coding books?

   _____

   A. What is the current price of the coding book?

   _____

2. Can you locate a vendor that sells an electronic version of the coding book?

   A. Can you determine the price of the software?

   _____

B. Is there a site that will let you use an electronic version for free or for a demo? If so, try looking up a few codes on the site. How easy is it? How accurate?

_____

_____

USING THE WEB WISELY

3. Referring to question 1 in Surfing The Net, use the criteria from Chapter 1, Using the Web Wisely, to evaluate the websites you found offering free electronic versions of the ICD-10-CM.

_____

_____

WEB SCAVENGER HUNT

4. Using your favorite browser, go to: www.cdc.gov/nchs/icd/icd10cm.htm#10update.

(1) Can you locate ICD-10-CM Guidelines?
(2) Are addenda to the ICD-10-CM available?

5. Using a search engine such as Google or Yahoo, search for the ICD-10.

(1) Are you able to purchase an ICD-10? If not, why not?

APPLYING CONCEPTS
ASSIGN ICD-10-CM CODES

1. Patient was seen in office and given blood tests. Doctor's diagnosis is group D hyperlipidema.

2. An astronaut returns to Earth and is diagnosed with dizziness due to the effects of weightlessness during the space mission.

3. A sixteen-year-old patient was seen in the office for a routine medical examination for a driver's license.

4. The patient suffered a first-degree sunburn of his upper body for the first time after spending the day at the beach.

5. A patient tested positive for mononucleosis and hepatitis.

6. The patient complains of hoarseness and, on examination, the doctor ruled out tonsillitis and strep throat.

7. A fifty-six-year-old woman had an anaphylactic reaction due to an accidental bee sting for the second time this year.

8. The patient has a history of a heart transplant and was seen in the office for a cold.

9. After examination, tests, and X-rays, the patient was diagnosed with infiltrative tuberculosis of the lung.

10. Patient is diagnosed with diabetes mellitus, type 1, with Kimmelstiel-Wilson disease.

11. A pregnant woman, in her third trimester, is diagnosed with gestational hypertension.

12. A healthy infant was given immunization for mumps, measles, and rubella.

13. A child was brought to the office after being poisoned by mistakenly drinking drain cleaner for the first time.

14. After a thorough examination, including appropriate tests, no disease was found although the patient expired.

15. The patient was diagnosed with intrapelvic Hodgkin's granuloma.

Procedural Coding: CPT AND HCPCS

Chapter 5

Learning Outcomes

After studying this chapter, you should be able to:

5.1 Explain the CPT code set.
5.2 Describe the organization of CPT.
5.3 Summarize the use of format and symbols in CPT.
5.4 Assign modifiers to CPT codes.
5.5 Apply the six steps for selecting CPT procedure codes to patient scenarios.
5.6 Explain how the key components are used in selecting CPT Evaluation and Management codes.
5.7 Explain the physical status modifiers and add-on codes used in the Anesthesia section of CPT Category I codes.
5.8 Differentiate between surgical packages and separate procedures in the Surgery section of CPT Category I codes.
5.9 State the purpose of the Radiology section of CPT Category I codes.
5.10 Code for laboratory panels in the Pathology and Laboratory section of CPT Category I codes.
5.11 Code for immunizations using Medicine section CPT Category I codes.
5.12 Contrast Category II and Category III codes.
5.13 Discuss the purpose of the HCPCS code set and its modifiers.

ASSISTED OUTLINING

Directions: *Read the chapter through one time. Then go back over the chapter and find the information required to complete the following outline of the chapter. Write the requested information directly in the spaces provided.*

1. List three uses for the CPT:

   (1)

   (2)

   (3)

5.1 Current Procedural Terminology, Fourth Edition (CPT)

1. Who owns and produces the CPT?

History

2. Give a brief history of the CPT.

3. Is the CPT used in other coding systems?

4. List three mandated uses of CPT codes.

   (1)   (3)

   (2)

Types of CPT Codes

5. List the three categories of CPT codes:

   (1)   (3)

   (2)

Category I Codes

6. How are CPT Category I codes written?

Category II Codes

7. How are CPT Category II codes written?

8. How are CPT Category II codes used?

Category III Codes

9. How are CPT Category III codes used?

10. How are CPT Category III codes written?

Updates

11. How are annual updates to the CPT determined?

12. When are annual updates available? Effective?

13. How often are vaccine and Category III codes updated?

14. When must new CPT codes be used? Is there a grace period?

5.2 Organization

1. List the six sections of CPT Category I procedure codes.

   (1)   (4)

   (2)   (5)

   (3)   (6)

The Index

2. What is the index and how is it used?

Main Terms and Modifying Terms

3. List the five types of main terms in the index:

   (1)   (4)

   (2)   (5)

   (3)

4. How are main terms printed? How are they listed? What is the use of subterms?

Code Ranges

5. What is the purpose of showing a range of codes?

Cross-References

6. Explain the use of the cross-reference *See* in the index.

The Main Text

7. Why must the code be located in the main text rather than selected from the index entry?

8. In what order are codes listed in the main text?

9. How is each of the headings used?

Guidelines

10. What are section guidelines? How are they used?

Unlisted Procedures

11. What is an unlisted procedure?

12. How are they used?

Special Reports

13. How are special reports used?

The Appendixes

14. Describe the content of the first appendix of CPT.

5.3 Format and Symbols

Format

Semicolons and Indentions

1. Explain how semicolons and indentions are used in the main text of the CPT.

Cross-References

2. How are cross-references listed?

Symbols for Changed Codes

3. What do the following symbols mean when they appear next to CPT codes?

(1) • (3) ► ◄

(2) ▲

Symbol for Add-On Codes

4. What is an add-on code? How are they identified in the main text?

Symbol for Moderate Sedation

5. What symbol is currently used for moderate sedation?

Symbol for FDA Approval Pending

6. What symbol is used for codes that are currently pending FDA approval?

Symbol for Resequenced Codes

7. How are resequenced codes listed in CPT?

5.4 CPT Modifiers

1. What is a modifier?

2. Can CPT codes from all six sections be used with a modifier? Give three examples.

(1) (3)

(2)

What Do Modifiers Mean?

3. What do modifiers mean?

4. Give six examples of situations when modifiers are used:

(1) (4)

(2) (5)

(3) (6)

Assigning Modifiers

5. How are modifiers shown/written?

6. How are multiple modifiers shown?

5.5 Coding Steps

1. List the six steps in the correct coding process.

(1)	**(4)**
(2)	**(5)**
(3)	**(6)**

Step 1 Review Complete Medical Documentation

2. How are the reported procedures and services determined?

Step 2 Abstract the Medical Procedures from the Visit Documentation

3. What is decided based on knowledge of CPT and of the payer's policies?

Step 3 Identify the Main Term for Each Procedure

4. What are main terms based on?

Step 4 Locate the Main Terms in the CPT Index

5. How are the procedures located in the CPT Index?

Step 5 Verify the Code in the CPT Main Index

6. How are the possible codes reviewed?

Step 6 Determine the Need for Modifiers

7. What may affect the use of modifiers?

5.6 Evaluation and Management Codes

1. What is coded using E/M codes?

2. Where are E/M codes listed in the CPT?

3. When and from where/whom did E/M codes originate?

Structure

4. What is the range of codes covering preventive medicine services in the E/M section of the CPT?

A New or Established Patient?

5. What is the abbreviation used for a new patient? An established patient?

6. Explain the distinction between a new patient and an established patient.

7. Explain the rules applied to professional services to designate a patient as an established patient.

A Consultation or a Referral?

8. What is the difference between a consultation and a referral?

E/M Code Selection

9. List the eight steps to be followed in selecting the correct E/M code.

(1)

(2)

(3)

(4)

(5)

(6)

(7)

(8)

Step 1 Determine the Category and Subcategory of Service Based on the Place of Service and the Patient's Status

10. What are the three key components used to select codes from this range of E/M codes?

(1)

(2)

(3)

11. What is the exception to the above guidelines?

Step 2 Determine the Extent of the History that Is Documented

12. How is historical information documented in a patient's medical record?

13. Define history of present illness.

14. List the fourteen body systems inventoried in the ROS.

(1)

(2)

(3)

(4)

(5)

(6)

(7)

(8)

(9)

(10)

(11)

(12)

(13)

(14)

15. What data are the focus of the PMH?

16. What types of medical events are included in family history?

17. What types of information are included in social history?

18. List and explain the four ways the PFSH is categorized.

    (1)   **(3)**

    (2)   **(4)**

Step 3 Determine the Extent of the Examination that Is Documented

19. List and explain the four ways the examination is categorized.

    (1)   **(3)**

    (2)   **(4)**

Step 4 Determine the Complexity of Medical Decision Making that Is Documented

20. List and explain the four ways the documented decision-making process is categorized.

    (1)   **(3)**

    (2)   **(4)**

Step 5 Analyze the Requirements to Report the Service Level

21. What are the three key components used to document the level of service?

    (1)   **(3)**

    (2)

Step 6 Verify the Service Level Based on the Nature of the Presenting Problem, Time, Counseling, and Care Coordination

22. List the two additional factors used in selecting correct E/M level codes.

    (1)   **(2)**

23. When and how is time used as the main criteria in selecting E/M codes?

Step 7 Verify that the Documentation Is Complete

24. Documentation must be sufficient to determine (1) _____ and (2) _____ .

Step 8 Assign the Code

25. In addition to assigning the code, what else is reviewed?

Documentation Guidelines for Evaluation and Management

26. Where can you locate guidelines for implementing E/M codes?

Office and Hospital Services

27. Define outpatient.

5.7 Anesthesia Codes

Structure

1. What are the sections and subsections of anesthesia codes?

Physical Status Modifiers

2. What two types of modifiers may be used with anesthesia codes?

(1)   (2)

3. List the six physical status modifiers used with anesthesia codes.

(1)   (4)

(2)   (5)

(3)   (6)

5.8 Surgery Codes

Surgical Package

1. List the six common services included in a surgery code.

(1)   (4)

(2)   (5)

(3)   (6)

2. What is a surgical package (also list another term used for the same meaning)?

3. Define global period.

4. What two types of services are not included in surgical package codes?

(1)   (2)

Separate Procedures

5. Explain what a separate procedure means in coding surgery.

Structure

6. How are the surgery subsections organized?

Modifiers

7. List and explain five of the modifiers commonly used to indicate special circumstances involved with surgical procedures.

(1)   (4)

(2)   (5)

(3)

Reporting Surgical Codes

8. What is fragmented billing?

Reporting Sequence

9. What is the proper sequence for listing surgery codes? Why?

5.9 Radiology Codes

1. List and explain the two parts of radiology procedures.

(1)   (2)

Unlisted Procedures and Special Reports

2. How are unlisted procedures reported in coding?

Contrast Material

3. Why are contrast materials sometimes administered?

4. What is the difference between *with contrast* and *without contrast*?

Structure and Modifiers

5. What is the difference in the structure of the radiology subsections and the radiation oncology subsections?

Reporting Radiology Codes

6. Where are most radiology services performed?

5.10 Pathology and Laboratory Codes

1. What four steps are included in a complete pathology or laboratory procedure?

(1)   (3)

(2)   (4)

Panels

   2. Define panels.

Unlisted Procedures and Special Reports

   3. How are unlisted procedures reported in coding?

Structure and Modifiers

   4. What are four ways procedures and services are listed in the index?

      (1)   (3)

      (2)   (4)

Reporting Pathology and Laboratory Codes

   5. What two organizations regulate performance of tests in the office?

      (1)   (2)

5.11 Medicine Codes

Structure and Modifiers

   1. How are medicine codes organized?

Reporting Medicine Codes

   2. How are immunizations and other injections coded?

5.12 Category II and Category III Codes

   1. Are Category II codes optional or mandatory?

   2. Category II codes are _____ digits followed by an _____ character.

   3. A Category III code is used if available instead of an _____ code.

5.13 HCPCS

   1. How is the HCPCS used?

   2. What is the Level I section of HCPCS?

   3. What is the purpose of Level II codes? Who is responsible for maintaining these codes?

Level II Codes

   4. How are the Level II codes written?

   5. What is durable medical equipment (DME)?

6. What section of HCPCS contains the codes for DME?

7. How has HIPAA affected the use of HCPCS?

Permanent versus Temporary Codes

8. Who makes up the CMS HCPCS Workgroup? What is its purpose?

Permanent Codes

9. Explain permanent national codes and how they are used.

10. If medical insurance specialists are unsure whether to use a miscellaneous code or a permanent national code, whom may they contact for help? How?

Temporary Codes

11. What are temporary national codes?

12. List the seven sections of temporary national codes and how they are used:

(1)   (5)

(2)   (6)

(3)   (7)

(4)

HCPCS Updates

13. When are permanent national codes changed? What is the process?

14. When are temporary national codes updated? What is the process?

15. Where can the medical billing specialist find the most current codes?

Coding Procedures

Coding Steps

16. What are the proper steps to use when coding HCPCS codes?

17. How are drugs listed in the HCPCS code book?

18. Do symbols in HCPCS mimic symbols used in CPT? Provide an example.

Reporting Quantities

19. How are quantities indicated when writing HCPCS codes?

HCPCS Modifiers

20. What do HCPCS Level II modifiers indicate?

21. How are HCPCS modifiers written?

22. List the three types of never events.

HCPCS Billing Procedures

Medicare/Medicaid Billing

23. What special consideration should the medical billing specialist take in coding for Medicare and Medicaid claims?

Private Payer Billing

24. Do all private payers use HCPCS codes? Must they use all the codes?

KEY TERMS
MATCHING

Match the definition with the correct term from the following word list.

A. add-on code	N. outpatient
B. bundled code	O. panel
C. Category I codes	P. physical status modifier
D. Category II codes	Q. primary procedure
E. Category III codes	R. professional component (PC)
F. consultation	S. never event
G. durable medical equipment	T. section guidelines
H. E/M codes	U. separate procedure
I. fragmented billing	V. special report
J. global period	W. surgical package
K. global surgery rule	X. technical component (TC)
L. key component	Y. unlisted procedure
M. modifier	Z. resequenced

(1) Situations when a policy never pays a provider.

(2) A type of code in which a group of related procedures are covered by a single code.

(3) These codes cover physicians' services that are performed to determine the best course for patient care.

(4) The grouping of related components prior to and after surgery under a single procedure code.

(5) The period of time that is covered for follow-up care.

(6) These codes have five digits (with no decimals) followed by a descriptor, which is a brief explanation of the procedure.

(7) Temporary codes for emerging technology, services, and procedures.

(8) A person seen in the provider's office or admitted to a health care facility, such as a hospital or nursing home, for a period of less than twenty-four hours.

(9) An examination by a second physician at the request of the patient's physician.

(10) A report that defines the nature, extent, and need for an unlisted procedure and describes the time, effort, and equipment necessary to provide it.

(11) A two-digit number that may be attached to five-digit procedure codes to indicate special circumstances when performing a procedure.

(12) Codes used to track performance measures.

(13) These codes, shown with a plus sign (+) next to the code, describe secondary procedures that are carried out in addition to a primary procedure.

(14) Certain laboratory tests that are customarily ordered together.

(15) When separate procedures are reported that should have been included under a bundled code.

SELF-QUIZ

1. Define each of the six sections of Category I codes.

(1)	**(4)**
(2)	**(5)**
(3)	**(6)**

2. How are each of the sections of Category I codes organized?

3. What key guidelines are followed for each of the sections of Category I codes? (Table 5.1)

4. Where are the E/M codes located in the CPT? Why?

5. Can any of the modifiers (as shown in Table 5.2 on page 155) be used with any code?

6. What does this symbol, •, in the CPT indicate?

7. What are physical status modifiers? When and why are they used?

8. List the six steps to correctly code procedures.

(1)   (4)

(2)   (5)

(3)   (6)

9. What is an unlisted procedure? When should an unlisted code be reported?

10. What does a range of codes, for example; Cervix biopsy. . . . . 57500, 57520; mean?

11. What types of products are included under durable medical equipment?

12. How are HCPCS codes written?

13. What organization created this coding system?

14. How often are these codes updated?

15. Explain the difference between permanent national codes and temporary national codes.

CRITICAL THINKING QUESTIONS

1. The code numbers are listed in the index. Why not code directly from it?

2. If a patient has bunions on both feet repaired during the same operation, why must you use modifier −50?

3. Why can't the provider simply code office visits by time spent with the patient?

4. While on a skiing vacation, you break your leg and are treated by a local provider. Upon returning home, your PCP removes the cast. Explain why or why not to use a bundled code.

5. Explain why a physical status modifier must be used with anesthesia codes.

6. What does the HCPCS workgroup do?

7. Explain the benefit of having HCPCS codes in addition to CPT codes.

8. Why would the medical billing specialist need to use HCPCS codes for patients other than those covered by Medicare?

9. How does an individual or group (such as a provider) get a HCPCS code added, changed, or deleted?

WEB ACTIVITIES

SURFING THE NET

1. Visit the American Health Information Management Association's website, www.ahima.org, to learn about coding certification.

   (1) Certification is offered in what areas?

   _____
   _____

   (2) What is the entry level coding certification?

   _____
   _____

   (3) What do you need to achieve this certification?

   _____
   _____

2. Visit the American Academy of Professional Coders' website, www.aapc.com, to learn about coding certification.

   (1) What certifications are offered?

   _____
   _____

   (2) What are the requirements for becoming certified?

   _____
   _____

3. Using the website of a local health care facility such as a hospital, search the employment database.

(1) Are there any employment opportunities in coding in your location?

_____

_____

(2) Are there any employment opportunities in medical records clerk or medical records management or health information technology (HIT)?

_____

_____

(3) What other similar job titles are used to list positions requiring skills in medical terminology and/or coding?

_____

_____

4. Using a search engine such as Google or Yahoo, locate the websites of each of the four durable medical equipment regional carriers.

(1) Which carrier serves your geographic area?

_____

_____

5. Using the website of one of the regional DME MAC carriers:

(1) What is EDI?

_____

_____

(2) How will EDI affect insurance claims?

_____

_____

(3) How can a practice implement EDI?

_____

_____

USING THE WEB WISELY

6. Using a job search engine such as Monster.com or CareerBuilder.com, search the employment database for your location using the term "medical coding."

(1) What employment opportunities in medical coding are available in your location?

_____

_____

(2) Are any opportunities in related fields, such as medical records clerk, found in your search?

_____

_____

(3) Are all listings for employment opportunities? If not, what is the purpose of the listing?

_____

_____

WEB SCAVENGER HUNT

7. Using your favorite browser, locate the AMA website for the CPT by searching for CPT or go to www.ama-assn.org.

(1) Search for "how a code becomes a code."

(a) Who maintains CPT?

(b) How are suggestions to add/change/delete a code reviewed?

(c) Who can suggest additons/changes/deletions?

8. Using the same search engine, search for CPT Category II codes.

(1) When were these codes released?

(2) List five additions/changes/deletions to the CPT.

(3) Compare these changed codes to the code listed in the current CPT.

APPLYING CONCEPTS
ASSIGN CPT CODES

1. Ian Schmidt, a 16-year-old patient, was seen in the office for a routine medical examination for a driver's license.

2. The patient was already under the effects of anesthesia when the blepharoplasty was cancelled.

3. An established patient presented in your office for incision and drainage of a foot bursa.

4. Nancy Noonan, a 72-year-old patient, received immunization for influenza.

5. Due to an occupational injury the patient had evisceration of ocular contents with implant. Two surgeons participated in the surgery.

6. The newborn boy had a simple clamp circumcision.

7. The patient complained of weight gain and night sweats. He was given a chest X-ray, two views, frontal and lateral.

8. In the OR, the patient had aortic valve replacement using a homograft valve with cardiopulmonary bypass. The patient has severe cardiovascular disease.

9. A 62-year-old male patient had a routine PSA test.

10. After an encounter with a raccoon, Jaleel received the first in a series of subcutaneous injections of human rabies immune globulin.

11. Kin Cheng presented to your office with an open wound on his leg and a possible fracture of his tibia while skateboarding. The MRI confirmed the diagnosis of open fracture, right tibia.

Using the tables on pages 81–82, select the appropriate E/M code for:

12. A 25-year-old patient visited the office for the first time with a chief complaint of sunburn on his back. The doctor took a brief history, performed a limited exam of the back, and there was little risk of complications and minimal treatment options.

13. Kathryn Matu was first seen in the office complaining of excessive weight gain in the body but thinning of her extremities and a "hump" on her upper back. She also noted a "moon-shaped" face, severe fatigue, irritability, nausea, and easy bruising. The patient was questioned in-depth about the onset and pace of weight gain and her eating and exercise habits. A thorough PFSH revealed no family history of similar symptoms and all body systems were also reviewed. She was examined thoroughly and given script for blood tests and asked to return in one week.

14. Using the chart note for Charlie Chevalier from Apply Concepts #4 in the chapter of the workbook on EHRs, HIPAA, and HITECH, select the appropriate E/M code.

15. Patient returned to the office with a complaint of a lump in her left breast. The doctor did a palpation exam and scheduled the patient for a mammogram and needle aspiration biopsy. Patient was given complete instructions on preparing for the biopsy procedure. She was also extensively educated as to the options, both surgical and non-surgical, pending intra-operative results of the biopsy. After much discussion, patient agreed to total mastectomy if the intra-operative biopsy results were adenocarcinoma.

ASSIGN HCPCS CODES

16. The patient needs a replacement bulb for his therapeutic light box.

17. A diabetic patient needed her left orthopedic shoe converted from a firm counter to a soft counter over the front of the foot.

18. A very large patient needs a special size wheelchair with extra seat depth and width.

19. A patient with a diagnosis of sleep apnea was dispensed a CPAP machine along with a face mask and accompanying headgear.

20. The patient received an injection of gamma globulin, IM, over 10 cc.

21. The patient plays in a senior softball league. The patient was treated with a four-pronged splint for a broken ring finger of the right hand after catching the softball.

22. A deaf patient received patient education via a sign language interpreter.

Decision Matrix for Established Patient Visit/Outpatient Procedure Codes Evaluation and Management Coding

Office Visit Established Patient or EP	History*	Examination*	Medical Decision Making*	EP Counseling and Coordination of Care	Nature of Presenting Problem	Time
99211					Minimal	5 minutes
99212	Problem focused	Problem focused	Straightforward	Consistent with nature of problem	Self-limited or minor	10 minutes
99213	Expanded problem focused	Expanded problem focused	Low complexity	Consistent with nature of problem	Low to moderate severity	15 minutes
99214	Detailed history	Detailed examination	Moderate complexity	Consistent with nature of problem	Moderate to high severity	25 minutes
99215	Comprehensive history	Comprehensive examination	High complexity	Consistent with nature of problem	Moderate to high severity	40 minutes

NOTE: In order to effectively utilize this matrix, a thorough understanding of the components and their definitions is required.

*Two of the three key components must meet or exceed the stated requirements to qualify for a particular level of service.

Decision Matrix for New Patient Visit/Outpatient Procedure Codes Evaluation and Management Coding

Office Visit New Patient or NP	History*	Examination*	Medical Decision Making*	Counseling and Coordination of Care	Nature of Presenting Problem	Time
99201	Problem focused	Problem focused	Straightforward	Consistent with nature of problem	Self-limited or minor	10 minutes
99202	Problem focused	Problem focused	Straightforward	Consistent with nature of problem	Low to moderate severity	20 minutes
99203	Detailed history	Detailed examination	Low complexity	Consistent with nature of problem	Moderate severity	30 minutes
99204	Comprehensive history	Comprehensive examination	Moderate complexity	Consistent with nature of problem	Moderate to high severity	45 minutes
99205	Comprehensive history	Comprehensive examination	High complexity	Consistent with nature of problem	Moderate to high severity	60 minutes

NOTE: In order to effectively utilize this matrix, a thorough understanding of the components and their definitions is required.

*All three key components must be met to qualify for a particular level of service.

23. The patient received a cardiokymography.

24. A licensed social worker from the state's child protection services department completed a full assessment of the child's family using a two-way audiovisual telecommunications system.

25. The patient presented at an urgent care center with gout and was given an injection of colchicine 2 mg.

Visit Charges and Compliant Billing

Chapter **6**

Learning Outcomes

After studying this chapter, you should be able to:

6.1 Explain the importance of code linkage on health care claims.
6.2 Describe the use and format of Medicare's Correct Coding Initiative (CCI) edits and medically unlikely edits (MUEs).
6.3 Discuss types of coding and billing errors.
6.4 Appraise major strategies that help ensure compliant billing.
6.5 Discuss the use of audit tools to verify code selection.
6.6 Describe the fee schedules that physicians create for their services.
6.7 Compare the methods for setting payer fee schedules.
6.8 Calculate RBRVS payments under the Medicare Fee Schedule.
6.9 Compare the calculation of payments for participating and nonparticipating providers, and describe how balance billing regulations affect the charges that are due from patients.
6.10 Differentiate between billing for covered versus noncovered services under a capitation schedule.
6.11 Outline the process of patient checkout.

ASSISTED OUTLINING

Directions: *Read the chapter through one time. Then go back over the chapter and find the information required to complete the following outline of the chapter. Write the requested information directly in the spaces provided.*

6.1 Compliant Billing

1. List four of the negative consequences of noncompliant billing.

(1)   (3)

(2)   (4)

2. What is code linkage?

6.2 Knowledge of Billing Rules

1. How can the medical billing specialist keep up with changes in payers' rules?

Medicare Regulations: The Correct Coding Initiative

2. Where can you locate the rules for Medicare billing?

3. What is the CCI?

4. How does the medical billing specialist learn about updates and changes?

5. What is an edit?

6. Give at least two examples of edits that are screened by Medicare.

   (1)   (2)

Organization of the CCI Edits

7. List the three types of edits.

   (1)   (3)

   (2)

8. Explain the column 1/column 2 code pairs edit.

9. Explain the mutually exclusive code edit.

10. Explain the modifier indicators edit.

Medically Unlikely Edits

11. What are medically unlikely edits (MUEs)?

Other Government Regulations

12. What is the OIG Work Plan?

13. How are OIG/CMS advisory opinions used?

14. What are the implications of hiring excluded parties?

Private Payer Regulations

15. How do private payers use edits? What are the guidelines? Where are they found?

6.3 Compliance Errors

1. List two reasons for compliance errors.

   (1)   (2)

Errors Relating to Code Linkage and Medical Necessity

2. What is meant by lack of medical necessity when claims are denied?

3. What three conditions must be met, in general, to support medical necessity?

(1)   (3)

(2)

Errors Relating to the Coding Process

4. List four of the eight typical coding problems that may cause rejected claims.

(1)   (3)

(2)   (4)

Errors Relating to the Billing Process

5. List five of the nine frequent errors related to the billing process.

(1)   (4)

(2)   (5)

(3)

6.4 Strategies for Compliance

Carefully Define Packaged Codes and Know Global Periods

1. What do many practices adopt to help decide what is included in a procedure?

Benchmark the Practice's E/M Codes with National Averages

2. How can a practice monitor upcoding?

Use Modifiers Appropriately

3. List the three modifiers that are especially important for compliant billing.

(1)   (3)

(2)

Modifier 25: Significant, Separately Identifiable Evaluation and Management Service by the Same Physician on the Same Day of the Procedure or Other Service

4. When should CPT modifier 25 be used?

Modifier 59: Distinct Procedural Service

5. When should CPT modifier 59 be used?

Modifier 91: Repeat Clinical Diagnostic Laboratory Test

6. When should CPT modifier 91 be used?

7. Under what circumstances should CPT modifier 91 not be used?

Be Clear on Professional Courtesy and Discounts to Uninsured/Low-Income Patients

Professional Courtesy

8. Define professional courtesy.

9. Why might a practice choose not to offer professional courtesy?

10. Routinely waiving which two types of payments violates the law?

(1)   (2)

11. List two ways physicians can clarify professional courtesy arrangements.

(1)   (2)

Discounts to Uninsured, Low-Income, and Self-Pay Patients

12. Is it legal for a practice to offer discounts to uninsured or low-income patients?

Maintain Compliant Job Reference Aids and Documentation Templates

13. What is a job reference aid and what is its purpose?

14. What is a documentation template and what is its purpose?

6.5 Audits

1. What is an audit? Who may perform an audit?

2. How is an audit conducted?

External Audits

3. Who performs an external audit? What is audited?

4. How are external audits conducted? When are they conducted?

Recovery Audit Contractor Initiative

5. What is the purpose of the Recovery Audit Contractor (RAC) initiative?

Internal Audits

6. What is the purpose of an internal audit? Who performs the audit?

7. What is the difference between a prospective audit and a retrospective audit?

Auditing Tools to Verify E/M Code Selection

8. How can the medical billing specialist or physician help to reduce subjective assigning of E/M codes?

9. How does the auditor help review E/M codes?

Auditing Example: Is It a Brief or Extended History of the Present Illness?

Selecting the Code

10. How is the extent of the patient's overall history described?

11. List the eight factors solicited in the HPI that are used when determining extent of history.

(1)	(5)
(2)	(6)
(3)	(7)
(4)	(8)

12. From the HPI, how is the extent calculated?

Auditing the Code Selection

13. How does the auditor verify the overall selection of E/M codes?

6.6 Physician Fees

1. Why is it important for medical insurance specialists to know as much as possible about their patients' insurance plans including billing rules, coverage guidelines, and patient payment responsibilities?

Sources for Physician Fee Schedules

2. Define usual fees.

How Physician Fees Are Set and Managed

3. How are physician fees determined?

4. How can the medical billing specialist help determine if the fees are correctly set?

6.7 Payer Fee Schedules

1. What are the two main methods payers use to establish rates? How are they calculated?

(1)   (2)

Usual, Customary, and Reasonable (UCR) Payment Structures

2. How are UCR fees determined?

Relative Value Scale (RVS)

3. How are RVS fees determined?

Resource-Based Relative Value Scale (RBRVS)

4. Who uses the RBRVS payment system? How is it calculated?

5. What are the three parts to an RBRVS fee:

   (1)   (3)

   (2)

6.8 Calculating RBRVS Payments

1. Where do physicians/practices get information on the yearly changes to fee schedules?

2. What are the five steps used to calculate a Medicare payment?

   (1)   (4)

   (2)   (5)

   (3)

6.9 Fee-Based Payment Methods

1. What are the three main methods payers use to pay providers?

   (1)   (3)

   (2)

Allowed Charges

2. What is an allowed charge? What other terms are used to mean the same?

3. What three things affect whether a provider actually receives the allowed charge?

   (1)   (3)

   (2)

4. Explain the allowed charge method.

5. Explain balance billing.

Contracted Fee Schedule

6. Explain how the contract fee schedule works.

6.10 Capitation

1. What is capitation?

Setting the Cap Rate

2. How is the cap rate determined?

3. How are noncovered services paid?

Provider Withholds

4. What is a provider withhold? How is it calculated?

KEY TERMS
MULTIPLE CHOICE

Circle the letter of the choice that best matches the definition or answers the question.

1. A formal examination or review of the practice's billing and/or accounting system.

   A. Internal audit
   B. External audit

   C. Compliance audit
   D. Audit

2. A private payer's or government investigator's review of selected records of a practice for compliance.

   A. Internal audit
   B. External audit

   C. Compliance audit
   D. Audit

3. These audits are routine and are performed periodically without a reason to think that a compliance problem exists.

   A. Internal audit
   B. External audit

   C. Compliance audit
   D. Audit

4. When a provider can bill the patient for the difference between a higher physician fee and a lower allowed charge.

   A. Balance billing
   B. Upcode

   C. Professional courtesy
   D. Capitation rate

5. The connection between a billed service and a diagnosis is called:

   A. Compliance audit
   B. OIG Fraud Alert

   C. Code linkage
   D. Assumptive coding

6. Medicare's national policy on correct coding, which is an ongoing process to standardize bundled codes and control improper coding that would lead to inappropriate payment for Medicare claims for physician services.

   A. OIG Fraud Alert

   B. Correct Coding Initiative (CCI)

   C. OIG Work Plan

   D. Relative Value Scale (RVS)

7. Using a procedure code that provides a higher reimbursement rate than the correct code.

   A. Assumptive coding

   B. Downcoding

   C. Upcoding

   D. Truncated coding

8. Using a lower level code that provides a lower reimbursement rate than the correct code.

   A. Assumptive coding

   B. Downcoding

   C. Upcoding

   D. Truncated coding

9. The choice of a physician to waive the charges for services to other physicians and their families.

   A. Professional courtesy

   B. Charge-based fee structure

   C. Provider withhold

   D. Write-off

10. Fees set by determining the percentage of the published fee ranges that payers will pay.

    A. Usual, customary, and reasonable fee

    B. Allowed charge

    C. Usual fee

    D. Medicare Physician Fee Schedule (MPFS)

SELF-QUIZ

1. Who implements the OIG work plan?

2. How is an internal audit different from an external audit?

3. Where does the medical insurance specialist locate the yearly conversion factor?

4. What is the main consequence of billing incorrectly?

5. What is code linkage?

CRITICAL THINKING QUESTIONS

1. Why should GPCIs be used when calculating payments?

2. Why does the conversion factor change each year?

3. How does balance billing benefit a practice?

4. How do private payers differ from Medicare in edits?

5. How do physicians set fees versus payers?

WEB ACTIVITIES

SURFING THE NET

1. Using a search engine such as Yahoo or Google, locate the CMS website concerning CCI edits.

   (1) Can you locate the website of an authorized provider of CCI editing software?

   _____

   _____

   (2) Can you locate the website of any other purveyors of editing software?

   _____

   _____

WEB SCAVENGER HUNT

1. Go to the website of the Office of Inspector General—http://oig.hhs.gov.

   (1) Can you locate information on the current year's or most recent year's OIG Work Plan?

      (a) What is the mission of the OIG?

   (2) Use the Search box to find the most current OIG Work Plan, and select a topic of interest to you from the Table of Contents.

      (a) Specifically what is being studied in that part of the current OIG Work Plan?

2. Go to the website regarding the Medicare Fee Schedule— www.cms.gov/apps/physician-fee-schedule/license-agreement.aspx. Accept the license agreement. Select the current year. Click the radio buttons next to Single HCPCS Code and Geographic Practice Cost Index. Click Next. Click the radio button next to Specific Locality. Click Next. Using the drop-down menu, select your locality, then click Submit.

   (1) What are the GPCIs for this location?

   (2) Repeat the steps choosing other locations. Are the GPCIs the same? Different? Why?

APPLYING CONCEPTS

Dr. Ellen Zook, an allergist, is a participating provider with Phoenix Care and Medicare. She is a nonparticipating provider with Cirrus Health. Patients frequently receive allergy scratch testing, CPT code 95004, and are charged $470. In addition, Dr. Zook charges $65 for the average established patient office visit, CPT code 99213, and $70 for the average new patient office visit, CPT code 99203.

1. Nils Hovik is an established patient and is covered by Phoenix Care through his employer. This specific group plan has neither copay nor coinsurance. He has met his deductible of $250 for this year. He visited Dr. Zook for itching and congestion. The encounter form listed two procedures: office visit and allergy scratch testing. Dr. Zook submitted a claim to Phoenix Care. The allowed charge under PhoenixPlus is $62 for 99213, $65 for 99203, and $477 for 95004.

   (1) What amount will Dr. Zook be reimbursed by Phoenix Care for each procedure? In total?

   (2) What amount, if any, will Dr. Zook write off for each procedure? In total?

   (3) What amount, if any, will be billed to Mr. Hovik for each procedure? In total?

2. Parminder Singh is an established patient also seen by Dr. Zook for an office visit and allergy scratch testing; however, she is insured by Cirrus Health. The allowed charge under Cirrus Health is $58 for 99213, $61 for 99203, and $420 for 95004.

   (1) What amount will Dr. Zook be reimbursed by Cirrus Health for each procedure? In total?

   (2) What amount, if any, will Dr. Zook write off for each procedure? In total?

   (3) What amount, if any, will be billed to Miss Singh for each procedure? In total?

3. Monica Salenski is a new patient covered by Cirrus Health. She was seen by Dr. Zook for an office visit and allergy scratch testing.

   (1) What amount will Dr. Zook be reimbursed by Cirrus Health for each procedure? In total?

   (2) What amount, if any, will Dr. Zook write off for each procedure? In total?

   (3) What amount, if any, will be billed to Miss Salenski for each procedure? In total?

4. Harris Theodore is a new patient covered by Medicare. He has met his yearly deductible; his coinsurance is 80-20. Medicare's allowed charge for 99213 is $52, for 99203 is $55, and for 95004 is $375. He was seen by Dr. Zook for an office visit and allergy scratch testing.

   (1) What amount will Dr. Zook be reimbursed by Medicare for each procedure? In total?

   (2) What amount, if any, will Dr. Zook write off for each procedure? In total?

   (3) What amount, if any, will be billed to Mr. Theodore for each procedure? In total?

Dr. Zook also accepts patients with PhoenixPlus, a non-Medicare PPO. New or established patients pay a copay of $15 for office visits. Dr. Zook's contract with PhoenixPlus includes a capitation schedule that sets capitation rates as follows:

Age/Gender	Rate
0-4 years, Female	$17.57
0-4 years, Male	$17.57
5-15 years, Female	$14.53
5-15 years, Male	$12.44
15-21 years, Female	$12.32
15-21 years, Male	$8.66

5. If Dr. Zook's practice has 208 children, aged 0 to 4 years F; and 156 children, aged 0 to 4 years M; as well as 93, F, aged 15 to 21, and 87, M, aged 15 to 21, what is the monthly capitation for each group? In total?

For the following questions, use the conversion factor of $41.53. The RVUs and GPCIs are as follows:

Description	Work RVU	Practice Expense RVU	Malpractice Expense RVU
Magnetic resonance angiography, pelvis, with or without contrast material, 72198	1.80	11.86	0.57
Screening mammography, bilateral (2-view film study of each breast), 77057	0.70	1.47	0.09
Fine needle aspiration; w/o imaging guidance, 10021	1.27	0.055	0.07
Polysomnography; sleep staging with 4 or more additional parameters of sleep, attended by technologist, 95810	3.53	16.92	0.47

Locality	Work GPCI	Practice Expense GPCI	Malpractice Expense GPCI
Macon, GA	1.01	1.089	0.966
Pierre, SD	1.0	0.876	0.365
Providence, RI	1.045	0.989	0.909

6. Using the tables shown, compute the anticipated payments for:

(1) A sleep study in Pierre, SD.

(2) A mammogram in Providence, RI.

(3) Fine needle aspiration in Macon, GA, and in Providence, RI.

(4) A magnetic resonance angiography in Macon, GA.

7. The director of coding/billing forwarded this memo to you, the medical insurance specialist, to help you plan for an internal audit.

Good Afternoon to All,

OIG today posts this report. As always, selecting the link immediately following the titles will take you directly to the full documents.

Use of Modifier 25 (OEI-07-03-00470)
www.oig.hhs.gov/oei/reports/oei-07-03-00470.pdf

OIG conducted this study to assess the extent to which use of modifier 25 meets program requirements. Modifier 25 is used to allow additional payment for evaluation and management (E/M) services performed by a provider on the same day as a procedure, as long as the E/M services are significant, separately identifiable, and above and beyond the usual preoperative and postoperative care associated with the procedure. OIG found that 35 percent of claims for E/M services allowed by Medicare in 2002 did not meet program requirements, resulting in $538 million in improper payments. Modifier 25 was also used unnecessarily on a large number of claims, and while such use may not lead to improper payments, it fails to meet program requirements. OIG recommends that CMS work with carriers to reduce the number of claims submitted using modifier 25 that do not meet program requirements, emphasize that providers must maintain appropriate documentation of both the E/M services and procedures, and remind providers that modifier 25 should only be used on claims for E/M services. CMS concurred with OIG's recommendations.

(1) What specific types of services will you audit?

(2) What specific codes or modifiers will you research?

(3) When is it acceptable to use modifier 25?

Chapter 7 Health Care Claim Preparation and Transmission

Learning Outcomes

After studying this chapter, you should be able to:

7.1 Distinguish between the electronic claim transaction and the paper claim form.

7.2 Discuss the content of the patient information section of the CMS-1500 claim.

7.3 Compare billing provider, pay-to provider, rendering provider, and referring provider.

7.4 Discuss the content of the physician or supplier information section of the CMS-1500 claim.

7.5 Explain the hierarchy of data elements on the HIPAA 837P claim.

7.6 Categorize data elements into the five sections of the HIPAA 837P claim transaction.

7.7 Evaluate the importance of checking claims prior to submission, even when using software.

7.8 Compare the three major methods of electronic claim transmission.

ASSISTED OUTLINING

Directions: Read the chapter through one time. Then go back over the chapter and find the information required to complete the following outline of the chapter. Write the requested information directly in the spaces provided.

7.1 Introduction to Health Care Claims

1. What format is mandated by HIPAA for electronic health care claims?

2. On what form is the HIPAA 837 claim form based?

Background

3. Which providers can continue to submit paper claims?

4. How have payers been affected by use of the HIPAA 837 claim form?

Claim Content

5. What organization is responsible for the development of both paper and electronic claim forms?

5010 Format and the CMS-1500

6. As of 2012, to what format must EDI transactions have moved?

7.2 Completing the CMS-1500 Claim: Patient Information Section

1. What do Item Numbers 1 through 13 on the CMS-1500 refer to? Where does this information come from?

2. What do Item Numbers 14 through 33 refer to? Where does this information come from?

Carrier Block

3. What information is listed in the carrier block?

Patient Information

4. What information do Item Numbers 1 through 13 of the CMS-1500 contain?

5. What is the importance of completing Item Numbers 10A through 10C?

6. What is the importance of Item Number 10D?

7. What is the insured's policy group number? What is the FECA number?

8. What is the importance of Item Number 12?

9. What is the importance of Item Number 13?

10. How frequently must SOF release forms be signed?

7.3 Types of Providers

1. List the four types of different providers that may need to be identified.

   (1)   (3)

   (2)   (4)

7.4 Completing the CMS-1500 Claim: Physician/Supplier Information Section

1. What information do Item Numbers 14 through 33 of the CMS-1500 contain?

Physician/Supplier Information

2. How should Item Number 17A be completed?

3. How does the medical billing specialist complete Item Number 19? Give an example.

4. What is the important billing consideration in completing Item Number 20?

5. How is Item Number 22 handled for Medicaid claims? For other payers?

6. What is service line information?

7. How many billing entries can be entered in Section 24?

8. What three indicators and codes may be used in Section 24? Where is information regarding HPCS codes entered in Section 24?

   (1)   (3)

   (2)

9. What information does POS provide?

10. How has information entered in Item Number 24C changed?

11. How is an unlisted procedure handled in Item Number 19?

12. What is the diagnosis pointer? How is it used?

13. How is information entered in Item Number 24I?

14. What information was previously entered in Item Number 24I, 24J, and 24K?

15. What is the difference between the information entered in Item Number 32 and Item Number 33?

A Note on Taxonomy Codes

16. What is a taxonomy code? Where is it used?

17. What are administrative code sets? How are they used?

7.5 The HIPAA 837P Claim

Use of PMPs

1. What three things are PMP vendors responsible for on HIPAA 837P claims?

    (1)   (3)

    (2)

Claim Organization

2. Give an example of a data element. How are they like Item Numbers?
3. What are the five major sections or levels of the claim?

    (1)   (4)

    (2)   (5)

    (3)

4. How are the five major sections of data elements organized? Must all data elements be submitted with each claim sent?
5. What are the four types of data elements?

    (1)   (3)

    (2)   (4)

7.6 Completing the HIPAA 837P Claim

Provider Information

1. List the four types of providers.

    (1)   (3)

    (2)   (4)

Subscriber Information

2. How is the term subscriber used on the HIPAA 837P claim form?

3. Who is a responsible party?

Claim Filing Indicator Code

4. What is a claim filing indicator code? When must they be used?

Relationship of Patient to Subscriber

5. What is an individual relationship code?

Other Data Elements

6. What are the three situational data elements? How are other data elements used?

(1)   (3)

(2)

Payer Information

7. Define destination payer.

8. What does the payer responsibility sequence number code identify? How is it used?

Claim Information

9. When would information about the rendering provider be supplied?

Claim Control Number

10. How is the claim control number used?

Claim Frequency Code

11. List the three types of claim frequency codes.

(1)   (3)

(2)

Diagnosis Codes

12. How many diagnosis codes may be entered on the HIPAA 837P claim form?

Claim Note

13. When is a claim note used?

Service Line Information

14. Does the HIPAA 837P have the same elements as the CMS-1500 at the service line level?

Diagnosis Code Pointers

15. How are diagnosis code pointers used on the HIPAA 837P claim form?

Line Item Control Number

16. How is the line item control number used?

Claim Attachments

17. Define claim attachment and give an example.

18. How are claim attachments for the HIPAA 837P claim form handled?

7.7 Checking Claims Before Transmission

1. How are claims checked before transmittal?

Clean Claims

2. What is a clean claim?

3. List four of the many errors that prevent claims from being processed by payers.

    (1)   (3)

    (2)   (4)

7.8 Clearinghouses and Claim Transmission

1. How does the office verify that a transaction has been received by the payer?
2. What is the most common method of submitting electronic media claims (EMC)?
3. List the three major methods of transmitting claims electronically.

    (1)   (3)

    (2)

Transmit Claims Directly

4. How does the provider transmit claims directly?

Use a Clearinghouse

5. How do clearinghouses help send HIPAA 837P claims?

Use Direct Data Entry (DDE)

6. Explain the DDE process.

7. If the medical billing specialist wants to know the status of a claim, what electronic transaction is completed?

8. What is a claim scrubber? How is it used?

KEY TERMS

MATCHING

Match the definition with the correct term from the following word list.

A. administrative code set	Q. HIPAA X12 837 Health Care Claim: Professional (837P)
B. billing provider	R. line item control number
C. carrier block	S. National Uniform Claim Committee (NUCC)
D. claim attachment	T. other ID number
E. claim control number	U. outside laboratory
F. claim filing indicator code	V. pay-to provider
G. claim frequency code (claim submission reason code)	W. place of service (POS) code
H. claim scrubber	X. primary provider identifier
I. clean claims	Y. qualifier
J. CMS-1500 claim	Z. referring provider
K. condition code	AA. rendering provider
L. data elements	BB. required data element
M. destination payer	CC. responsible party
N. 5010 version	DD. service line information
O. HIPAA X12 276/277 Health Care Claim Status Inquiry/Response	EE. situational data element
P. individual relationship code	FF. subscriber
	GG. taxonomy code

1. As of 2012, the format EDI transactions must use

2. The organization or person transmitting the claim to the payer, usually a billing service or clearinghouse

3. A 20-character identifier assigned by the sender that is unique for each claim

4. An editing software program that makes sure that all required fields are filled and that only valid codes are used, and performs other checks

5. The organization that determines the content of both paper and electronic claims

6. Those claims, without errors, that are accepted for adjudication by payers

7. A code required to specify the patient's relationship to the subscriber when the patient and the subscriber are not the same person

8. A ten-digit number that stands for a physician's medical specialty

9. Alternate term for insured/guarantor/policyholder

10. Receives the payment from the insurance carrier

11. A paper claim form containing a possible 33 boxes of information about the patient and/or insured, provider, and services provided

12. The physician who provides the patient's treatment

13. An entity or person other than the subscriber or patient who has financial responsibility for the bill

14. The portion of the claim that reports the procedures/services performed for the patient

15. The payer to whom the claim is going to be sent

SELF-QUIZ

1. Give three examples of data elements used in the HIPAA 837P claim.

   (1)   (3)

   (2)

2. What cannot be used as the claim control number?

3. Explain how the diagnosis pointer is used on the CMS-1500.

4. What is the difference between using a clearinghouse and DDE?

5. What is the difference between a line item control number and a claim control number?

CRITICAL THINKING QUESTIONS

1. Explain the importance in terms of billing of completing Item Numbers 10A through 10D on the CMS-1500.

2. List three benefits of using electronic claim transmission.

   (1)   (3)

   (2)

3. If the patient chooses to pay by debit or credit card, why is the amount not charged immediately?

4. How does a PMP make claim preparation and submission easier?

5. The CMS-1500 and the HIPAA 837P do not report the exact same information or use the same sequence of information. Why do you think there is a difference? Give examples.

WEB ACTIVITIES

SURFING THE NET

1. Go to the website for the National Uniform Claim Committee, www.nucc.org. Click on or search for CMS-1500. (This is a PDF file.)

   A. Click on 1500 Claim Form, Table of Changes.

   (1) Are there any current changes to the CMS-1500 form? If so, list them.

   _____

   _____

   B. Click on Resources.

   (1) What types of resources are available from this website?

   _____

   _____

   C. Click on the link to the American Dental Association. In the search box, type *claim form.*

   (1) How is the ADA dental claim form different from the CMS-1500?

   _____

   _____

   (2) How are the ADA dental claim form and the CMS-1500 similar?

   _____

   _____

   (3) Can the two claim forms be used interchangeably? Why or why not?

   _____

   _____

USING THE WEB WISELY

1. Using a search engine such as Google or Yahoo, search for POS codes.

   A. What are other meanings for the abbreviation POS?

   _____

   _____

   B. Can you locate a website, other than CMS, that offers POS codes for use in preparing claims?

   _____

   _____

WEB SCAVENGER HUNT

1. Go to the website for Place of Service codes,
   www.cms.gov/Medicare/Coding/place-of-service-codes/.
   A. Find the POS Database in the document.
      (1) What is the POS code for a mass immunization clinic?
      (2) What is the POS code for an independent laboratory?
      (3) What is the POS code for a hospital emergency room?

USING MATH IN THE MEDICAL OFFICE

To complete service line information entries on claims, the medical billing specialist must calculate units of measure.

1. After an amputation above the knee, the patient was fitted with a prosthetic sock, HCPCS code L8480. He also received six additional socks for daily wearing. How would this be entered on the service line in Item Number 24?

2. The anesthesia for an operative procedure lasted 1 hour and 45 minutes. Complete the calculation necessary to enter the minutes of anesthesia in Item Number 24G on the CMS-1500.

3. An established patient was seen three times at the nursing home where she resides. The CPT code used is 99334. How would this be entered on the service line in Item Number 24?

4. A patient with a lung condition was dispensed 28 vials of Albuterol 0.5mg (HCPCS code J7620) for use at home with a nebulizer. Complete the calculation necessary to enter the unit reported for service line information.

5. The patient, a vacationer, was seen once in the office for treatment of sunburn. What unit is entered in Item Number 24G?

APPLYING CONCEPTS

1. The patient was a passenger in a school bus that was involved in a traffic accident in your state. How would the medical insurance specialist complete Item Numbers 10A through 10C?

```
10. IS PATIENT'S CONDITION RELATED TO:


a. EMPLOYMENT? (CURRENT OR PREVIOUS)
        ☐ YES      ☐ NO
b. AUTO ACCIDENT?
                        PLACE (State)
        ☐ YES      ☐ NO ⌊___⌋
c. OTHER ACCIDENT?
        ☐ YES      ☐ NO
```

Note: Use the blank CMS-1500 (02/12) form at the back of the book to complete questions 2, 3, and 4.

2. Using the patient information in Case 7.2, complete Item Numbers 1 through 13 of the CMS-1500 (02/12).

3. Using the patient information in Case 7.3, complete Item Numbers 1 through 13 of the CMS-1500 (02/12).

4. Using the patient information in Case 7.4, complete Item Numbers 14 through 33 of the CMS-1500 (02/12). You may also need to consult other pages in this chapter to complete Item Number 24.

5. When filing a HIPAA 837P claim, it is important that all data elements necessary for the processing and adjudication of a claim are included in the electronic transmission of data. Using the information in Case 7.3 as well as Table 7.4, HIPAA Data Elements, can the Pay-to Provider section of the claim be completed? Why or why not?

Private Payers/BlueCross BlueShield

Chapter 8

Learning Outcomes

After studying this chapter, you should be able to:

8.1 Compare employer-sponsored and self-funded health plans.

8.2 Describe the major features of group health plans regarding eligibility, portability, and required coverage.

8.3 Discuss provider payment under the various private payer plans.

8.4 Contrast health reimbursement accounts, health savings accounts, and flexible savings (spending) accounts.

8.5 Discuss the major private payers.

8.6 Analyze the purpose of the five main parts of participation contracts.

8.7 Describe the information needed to collect copayments and bill for surgical procedures under contracted plans.

8.8 Discuss the use of plan summary grids.

8.9 Prepare accurate private payer claims.

8.10 Explain how to manage billing for capitated services.

ASSISTED OUTLINING

Directions: Read the chapter through one time. Then go back over the chapter and find the information required to complete the following outline of the chapter. Write the requested information directly in the spaces provided.

8.1 Private Insurance

1. Who may be covered under private insurance?

Employer-Sponsored Medical Insurance

2. What is a rider?

3. What is meant by "carve out" benefits? Give two examples.

(1)   (2)

4. Define open enrollment period.

5. How are employer-sponsored group health plans regulated?

Federal Employees Health Benefits Program

6. What is the Federal Employees Health Benefits program? Who is covered? How many health plans are available? Who administers this benefit? Who adjudicates claims?

Self-Funded Health Plans

7. Explain how a self-funded health plan works.

8. How are self-funded health plans regulated?

9. How are tasks such as claims processing often handled by self-funded health plans?

Individual Health Plans

10. What is an individual health plan? What is normally covered? Who are often the purchasers?

8.2 Features of Group Health Plans

1. What is a cafeteria plan?

2. What are the tax benefits of group health plans?

Eligibility for Benefits

3. List three of the typical eligibility rules of group health plans.

(1)   (3)

(2)

Waiting Period

4. Explain how a typical waiting plan works.

Late Enrollees

5. What is a late enrollee?

Premiums and Deductibles

6. What is the difference between an individual deductible and a family deductible?

Benefit Limits

7. Explain lifetime limits on benefits.

Tiered Networks

8. What is the purpose of a tiered network?

9. Define formulary.

Portability and Required Coverage

COBRA

10. What is COBRA and how does it benefit patients?

HIPAA

11. How does HIPAA help to regulate COBRA rules on preexisting conditions? Do any other laws affect preexisting conditions?

12. What is creditable coverage and what is the process to use this coverage?

13. What, if any, conditions are exempt from preexisting condition rules?

Other Federally Guaranteed Insurance Provisions

14. List the four other federal laws that govern private insurance coverage.

(1)   (3)

(2)   (4)

8.3 Types of Private Payers

1. List the seven types of private payer plans.

(1)   (5)

(2)   (6)

(3)   (7)

(4)

2. How are private payers regulated?

Preferred Provider Organizations

3. How is a PPO created?

4. How are a PPO's providers paid?

5. What must patients usually pay under a PPO for in-network and out-of-network providers?

6. What are two advantages of a PPO?

(1)   (2)

Health Maintenance Organizations

7. How are HMOs licensed? How do they operate?

8. What is the difference between an open-panel HMO and a closed-panel HMO?

9. What is "first dollar coverage?"

Staff Model

10. List the three main components of a staff model HMO.

(1)   **(3)**

(2)

Group (Network) Model

11. How is the group (network) model HMO different from the staff model HMO?

12. What is subcapitation?

13. What is an EOC option?

Independent Practice Association Model

14. Explain how an IPA operates.

Point-of-Service (POS) Plans

15. Explain how a POS plan charges for care in- and out-of-network.

Indemnity Plans

16. What is required of indemnity plans?

8.4 Consumer-Driven Health Plans (CDHP)

1. What two components are parts of a consumer-driven health plan? What does each cover?

(1)   **(2)**

2. What is the goal of CDHPs? How is this goal to be achieved?

The High-Deductible Health Plan

3. What is the plan's deductible? What is not included in the deductible?

The Funding Options

4. What are the three types of CDHP funding options?

    (1)   (3)

    (2)

Health Reimbursement Accounts (HRA)

5. How does an HRA work? What happens to funds left in the account at the end of the year?

Health Savings Accounts (HSA)

6. How were HSAs permitted? When were they first established?

7. How do employers encourage HSAs?

8. How much can be saved for an HSA?

9. Who holds the monies placed in the HSA account?

10. How are HSA funds different from HRA funds?

Flexible Savings (Spending) Accounts (FSA)

11. What is a FSA? How is it funded and used?

12. How does the patient receive the funds from the FSA?

13. What is the major disadvantage of a FSA?

Billing Under Consumer-Driven Health Plans

14. How can CDHPs reduce cash flow?

15. List the four steps for reimbursement in a CDHP:

    (1)   (3)

    (2)   (4)

16. How does an integrated CDHP help reimbursement?

17. How can debit and credit cards help in reimbursement?

18. List three factors that help avoid uncollectible accounts under CDHPs.

    (1)   (3)

    (2)

8.5 Major Private Payers and the BlueCross BlueShield Association

1. List five types of insurance services that are supplied by private payers.

(1)   (4)

(2)   (5)

(3)

Major Payers and Accrediting Groups

2. List four of the major national payers.

(1)   (3)

(2)   (4)

3. List the five major accrediting agencies and what they do.

(1)   (4)

(2)   (5)

(3)

4. How is the BlueCross BlueShield Association different from a major national payer?

BlueCross BlueShield Association

5. What is the BCBS Association? What types of insurance plans does it offer?

6. What is BCBS' P4P program?

Subscriber Identification Card

7. List the twelve items included on the BCBS identification card.

(1)   (7)

(2)   (8)

(3)   (9)

(4)   (10)

(5)   (11)

(6)   (12)

Types of Plans

8. What are the typical features of a BCBS indemnity plan?

9. Describe the three most common managed care programs offered by BCBS.

(1)   (3)

(2)

BlueCard Program

10. What is the BlueCard program?

11. List the five steps for provider reimbursement of the BlueCard program.

(1)   (4)

(2)   (5)

(3)

Flexible Blue Plan

12. What CDHPs does BCBS offer?

8.6 Participation Contracts

1. What is the primary factor that providers consider when deciding to participate in health plans?

Contract Provisions

2. What is the major question to be answered before a practice decides to participate with a particular health plan?

3. List the five main parts of a participation contract.

(1)   (4)

(2)   (5)

(3)

Introductory Section

4. List three important pieces of information provided in the introduction section of a participation contract.

(1)   (3)

(2)

Contract Purpose and Covered Medical Services

5. List three important pieces of information provided in the contract purpose and covered medical services section of a participation contract.

(1)   (3)

(2)

Physician's Responsibilities

6. List the six responsibilities of the physician under the participation contract.

(1)   (4)

(2)   (5)

(3)   (6)

7. List the four obligations of the managed care plan.

(1)   (3)

(2)   (4)

8. What is a stop-loss provision?

9. What do the compensation and billing guidelines cover?

8.7 Interpreting Compensation and Billing Guidelines

1. How may allowed amounts be calculated?

Compiling Billing Data

2. What is the purpose of billing the normal fee and then writing off the difference?

Billing for No-Shows

3. How may the physician bill for no shows?

Collecting Copayments

4. List three variables that affect the payment of copays.

(1)   (3)

(2)

5. List two ways copays may be handled.

(1)   (2)

6. Is it acceptable for a practice to routinely waive copays and deductibles?

Avoiding Silent PPOs

7. What is a silent PPO? Why is it important to know for the medical billing specialist?

Billing Surgical Procedures

8. How are emergency surgery cases typically approved?

9. What is elective surgery? How does the medical billing specialist know if the proposed procedure is covered?

10. What is a URO?

8.8 Private Payer Billing Management: Plan Summary Grids

1. List four questions the medical billing specialist should be able to answer about an insurance plan.

   (1)   (3)

   (2)   (4)

2. What is a plan summary grid? What key information should it include?

3. Explain the difference between a consult and a referral.

8.9 Preparing Correct Claims

1. List the first seven steps in the standard medical billing cycle.

   (1)   (5)

   (2)   (6)

   (3)   (7)

   (4)

2. What is the key step in verifying coverage?

3. What is a repricer? What is a negative of using a repricer?

4. List four main areas to check when preparing claims.

   (1)   (3)

   (2)   (4)

Communications with Payers

5. How can a practice establish effective communications with payers?

8.10 Capitation Management

Patient Eligibility

1. What is a monthly enrollment list? What other names are used for it?

Referral Requirements

2. Can a patient be balance-billed if the patient self-refers to a nonparticipating provider?

Encounter Reports and Claim Write-offs

3. What accounting problem could occur in billing for capitated payments?

Billing for Excluded Services

4. How are excluded services billed?

KEY TERMS

DEFINITIONS

Define the following terms:

1. Discounted fee-for-service

2. Episode of care (EOC) option

3. Flexible savings account (FSA)

4. Health reimbursement account (HRA)

5. Health savings account (HSA)

6. High deductible health plan (HDHP)

7. Independent practice association (IPA)

8. Late enrollee

9. Precertification

10. Stop-loss provision

SELF-QUIZ

1. How does COBRA affect employees?

2. What are the two components of CDHPs?

    (1)   (2)

3. List the seven steps in the medical billing cycle.

    (1)   (5)

    (2)   (6)

    (3)   (7)

    (4)

4. How are plan summary grids useful to the medical billing specialist?

5. What is the URO's purpose?

CRITICAL THINKING QUESTIONS

1. Explain the difference between HRA, HSA, and FSA.

2. How does the BCBS Association operate?

3. Why is it important to receive a monthly enrollment list from a health plan?

4. What are write-offs and how do they affect the practice's accounting system?

5. How are group health plans and TPAs governed by HIPAA?

WEB ACTIVITIES

USING THE WEB WISELY

1. Go to www.naic.org/state_web_map.htm.

    A. Who is NAIC?

    _____

    _____

    B. In your opinion, is this website objective?

    _____

    _____

    C. When was this site last updated?

    _____

    _____

2. Locate the website of Department of Insurance in your state.

    A. Where is this organization located?

    _____

    _____

    B. Who is the current head of this organization?

    _____

    _____

C. What is the purpose of your state's Department of Insurance?

_____

_____

D. How can the medical billing specialist contact the department?

_____

_____

WEB SCAVENGER HUNT

1. Go to www.bcbs.com/. Locate the website of a BCBS member plan in your state/region/city.

  A. What is the name of the member plan?

  _____

  _____

  B. What is the geographic area of coverage?

  _____

  _____

  C. How can the medical billing specialist contact this plan?

  _____

  _____

  D. What types of policies/plans are offered by this member plan?

  _____

  _____

  E. Can individuals purchase policies?

  _____

  _____

2. Locate a member plan in another state/region/city.

  A. What is the name of the member plan?

  _____

  _____

  B. What is the geographic area of coverage?

  _____

  _____

  C. How can the medical billing specialist contact this plan?

  _____

  _____

  D. What types of policies/plans are offered by this member plan?

  _____

  _____

E. Can individuals purchase policies?

_____

_____

F. How do this plan's offerings differ from those in your area's member plan?

_____

_____

_____

APPLYING CONCEPTS

1. Kin Cheng is covered by Golden Sun PPO and has a copay of $15. Golden Sun PPO pays a discounted fee-for-service of 80 percent of the provider's usual charge. For his last office visit, the charges totaled $143.50. What amount is paid to the provider? By whom?

2. Barbara Saxton required a chest X-ray, two views, CPT code 71020. The provider charges $164. Her provider participates in the local BCBS POS plan. The POS plan reimburses using a contracted fee schedule; the fee for CPT code 71020 is $120. What amount is paid to the provider? What amount is billed to the patient?

3. Benton Button's employer provides an HSA to accompany his HDHP. His deductible is $1,500 per year (which is not yet met) and coinsurance is 75-25. Benton may seek treatment from any provider. He is contemplating necessary surgery with three different providers. Provider X charges $11,294; Provider Y charges $10,960; and Provider Z charges $11,318. Providers X and Y offer as an additional incentive a 5 percent discount for payment up front.

   A. What is the charge for each provider?

   B. What amount will Benton be required to pay?

For these questions, refer to Figure 8.2 in your textbook.

• Iris and Hector Guzman and their children are new patients covered by the PPO. Their copayment is $10 for office visits. They have an annual deductible of $500 for out-of-network charges as well as coinsurance of 80-20.

4. Iris takes her three children, ages 5 months, 3 years, and 8 years, for routine well-child visits to a network provider. The infant and 3-year-old receive immunizations. What amount will the Guzmans be required to pay?

5. Iris, age 35, also receives a physical and screening mammogram from a network provider. What amount will the Guzmans be required to pay?

6. While on vacation in another state, the 8-year-old fell. He was seen in a walk-in medical center; charges were $85. The physician felt that he may have a broken wrist and also ordered an X-ray; charges were $120. The X-ray showed a fracture and a cast was applied to the child's wrist; charges were $165. What is the total amount the Guzmans will be required to pay?

7. After returning home from vacation, the child's cast is removed. He goes to outpatient physical therapy with a network provider for eight visits. What is the total amount the Guzmans will be required to pay?

8. Hector has had a persistent respiratory condition for several months. He is seen by the physician for an office visit. The physician also orders a chest X-ray that is not clear enough. The physician then orders a CAT scan. What is the total amount the Guzmans will be required to pay?

9. Hector wishes to get a second opinion and so visits a physician who is not in the PPO network. This physician also orders a CAT scan. Total charges were $70 for office visit and $535 for CAT scan. What is the total amount the Guzmans will be required to pay?

10. What is the total amount paid by the Guzmans for health care so far this year?

Medicare

Chapter 9

Learning Outcomes

After studying this chapter, you should be able to:

9.1 List the eligibility requirements for Medicare program coverage.

9.2 Differentiate among Medicare Part A, Part B, Part C, and Part D.

9.3 Contrast the types of medical and preventive services that are covered or excluded under Medicare Part B.

9.4 Apply the process that is followed to assist a patient in completing an ABN form correctly.

9.5 Calculate fees for nonparticipating physicians when they do and do not accept assignment.

9.6 Outline the features of the Original Medicare Plan.

9.7 Discuss the features and coverage offered under Medicare Advantage plans.

9.8 Explain the coverage that Medigap plans offer.

9.9 Discuss the Medicare, Medical Review (MR), recovery auditor, and ZPIC programs.

9.10 Prepare accurate Medicare primary claims.

ASSISTED OUTLINING

Directions: Read the chapter through one time. Then go back over the chapter and find the information required to complete the following outline of the chapter. Write the requested information directly in the spaces provided.

1. When and how was Medicare established? Who manages Medicare?

9.1 Eligibility for Medicare

1. What does defined benefit program mean?

2. List Medicare's six eligible beneficiary categories.

(1)   (4)

(2)   (5)

(3)   (6)

9.2 The Medicare Program

Medicare Part A

1. What is covered under Medicare Part A? What is another name for Medicare Part A?

2. Who is covered under Medicare Part A? How do beneficiaries enroll? What is the cost?

Medicare Part B

3. What is covered under Medicare Part B?

4. Who is covered under Medicare Part B?

5. How do participants enroll in Medicare Part B?

6. What is the cost of Medicare Part B?

7. What two plans are available under Medicare Part B?

Medicare Part C

8. How is Medicare Part C provided?

9. How was Medicare Part C previously known?

10. Who is eligible for Medicare Part C?

Medicare Part D

11. What is covered under Medicare Part D?

12. Who offers this service?

13. Explain the difference between the two types of plans.

9.3 Medicare Coverage and Benefits

1. What information is included on the Medicare card?

2. How is the HICN usually written?

3. What do the prefixes A, MA, WA, or WD indicate?

Medicare Claim Processing

4. What does a fiscal intermediary do?

5. What does a carrier/regional contractor do?

6. What is the new term Medicare uses to mean carrier?

7. Where is Medicare's main office located? Are there any other offices?

8. What are the four areas covered by the field office Consortia?

(1)   (3)

(2)   (4)

Medical Services and Other Services

9. What four main things are covered under Medicare Part B?

10. How are covered medical services paid for by the patient using a participating provider?

11. How are covered clinical laboratory services paid for by the patient using a participating provider?

12. How are covered home health care services paid for by the patient using a participating provider?

13. How are covered outpatient hospital services paid for by the patient using a participating provider?

14. How are covered blood services paid for by the patient using a participating provider?

15. List ten of the many other products and services covered under Part B.

(1)   (6)

(2)   (7)

(3)   (8)

(4)   (9)

(5)   (10)

Preventive Services

16. What preventive services are covered under Part B for qualified individuals?

17. Define a screening service.

Excluded Services and not Medically Necessary Services

18. How is Medicare coverage determined?

19. What are excluded services?

20. There are at least fifteen types of excluded services in Medicare. List seven.

(1)   (5)

(2)   (6)

(3)   (7)

(4)

21. Explain the difference between services not covered and services classified as not medically necessary by Medicare.

22. List three reasons for denial of medical necessity.

(1)   (3)

(2)

9.4 Medicare Participating Providers

1. When can physicians choose to participate or not participate in Medicare?

2. What is meant by participating physician under Medicare?

3. How does CMS ensure that enrolled providers are qualified?

4. What is the Medicare Learning Network (MLN)?

Incentives

5. What incentives are offered by Medicare to encourage participation?

6. What is the Physician Quality Reporting System (PQRS)?

Payments

7. How are payments handled for participating providers?

8. How was the MPFS developed?

Advance Beneficiary Notice (ABN)

9. How can a participating physician bill for services deemed not reasonable and necessary by Medicare?

10. How does the provider keep up-to-date about the medical necessity of specific services?

Mandatory ABNs

11. How is the patient informed if the specific service is deemed not reasonable or necessary?

12. What is the purpose of an ABN?

Voluntary ABNs

13. Give an example of an excluded service.

How To Complete the ABN

14. List the five sections of the ABN.

(1)   (4)

(2)   (5)

(3)

Modifiers for ABNs

15. How are noncovered Medicare services identified on claims?

9.5 Nonparticipating Providers

1. How do nonparticipating physicians accept assignment?

Payment Under Acceptance of Assignment

2. How are nonparticipating providers who accept assignment paid by Medicare?

Payment for Unassigned Claims: The Limiting Charge

3. What is the purpose of CLCCP?

4. What is a limiting charge?

5. What is excluded from limiting charges?

6. How are nonassigned claims billed?

9.6 Original Medicare Plan

1. What is another name for Medicare's Original Medicare Plan?

2. What are three key features of the Original Medicare Plan?

(1)   (3)

(2)

3. What is the patient's responsibility under the Original Medicare Plan?

4. What is the purpose of the MSN and how is it presented?

5. Is it a good idea to routinely waive patient payments such as deductibles? Why or why not?

9.7 Medicare Advantage Plans

1. What is another name for the Medicare Advantage Plans?

2. List three types of MAO plans. What do they cover?

(1)   (3)

(2)

Medicare Coordinated Care Plans

3. What is included in Medicare CCPs?

4. Who operates Medicare CCPs?

5. How does Medicare control utilization of CCPs?

6. What types of plans are included in Medicare's CCP plans?

(1)   (4)

(2)   (5)

(3)

7. List the key features of each type of Medicare CCP plan.

(1)   (4)

(2)   (5)

(3)

8. What services must be or may be offered by Medicare CCPs?

Medicare Private Fee-for-Service (PFFS)

9. What are the two key features of the Medicare PFFS plans?

(1)   (2)

Medical Savings Accounts

10. How does a Medicare Medical Savings Account work?

9.8 Additional Coverage Options

1. How do individuals obtain Medigap and/or supplemental insurance?

Medigap Plans

2. What is the purpose of Medigap insurance?

3. What type of Medicare patients can purchase Medigap policies?

4. Who pays for Medigap policies? How many are available? What are the premiums?

5. How are Medigap claims processed?

Supplemental Insurance

6. What is supplemental insurance?

9.9 Medicare Billing and Compliance

CCI Edits and Global Surgical Packages

1. What code set is used to code services for Medicare?

2. What is Medicare's CCI? How often is it updated?

3. What are the two major guidelines to be followed for correct global surgery package billing?

Consultation Codes: Noncompliant Billing

4. What modifier identifies the physician who oversees a patient's care from other physicians and who may be furnishing specialty care?

Timely Filing

5. What were the timely filing guidelines for Medicare?

Medicare Integrity Program

6. What is the purpose of the Medicare Integrity Program?

7. To what are the initiatives of the MIP related?

Medical Review Program

8. What is Medicare's Medical Review Program?

9. List and explain three types of Medicare medical reviews.

   (1)   (3)

   (2)

10. What steps should the medical billing specialist take for a comprehensive medical review?

Recovery Auditor Program

11. What is the objective of the RAC program?

Zone Program Integrity Contractors

12. What are Zone Program Integrity Contractors?

Duplicate Claims

13. What is a duplicate claim?

14. How can duplicate claims be avoided?

Split Billing

15. What is split billing?

Clinical Laboratory Improvement Amendments

16. How is lab work regulated?

17. How can Medicare providers perform waived tests?

18. How are CLIA-waived tests billed?

Incident-to Billing

19. Explain incident-to billing.

Roster Billing

20. What is roster billing?

21. What are three guidelines to follow when coding for roster billing for Medicare?

(1)   (3)

(2)

9.10 Preparing Primary Medicare Claims

1. Who is excluded from mandatory electronic billing under HIPAA?

2. What is the process for submitting claims including documentation to Medicare?

Medicare Required Data Elements on the HIPAA 837P Claim

Information in the Notes Segment

3. What is reported in the Notes Segment of the HIPAA 837P?

Diagnosis Codes

4. Are diagnosis codes required on the HIPAA 837P?

Medicare Assignment Code

5. What are the four Medicare assignment codes? What do they indicate?

(1)   (3)

(2)   (4)

Insurance Type Code

6. When is an insurance type code used?

7. List five of the fifteen insurance type codes.

(1)   (4)

(2)   (5)

(3)

Assumed Care Date/Relinquished Care Date

8. When is the assumed care date/relinquished care date used?

CMS-1500 Claim Completion

9. What procedure is followed if a patient is covered by both Medicare and a Medigap plan?

KEY TERMS

MULTIPLE CHOICE

Circle the letter of the choice that best matches the definition or answers the question.

1. Entities contracted by Medicare to handle claims and related functions for both Parts A and B are known as:

   A. Fiscal intermediaries   C. Third-party payers
   B. MACs   D. HMOs

2. MAC stands for:

   A. Medicare administrative contractor   C. Modernization Act cap
   B. Medicare Advantage C   D. Medicare (Part) A Consortium

3. Physicians may not charge a Medicare patient more than 115 percent of the amount listed in the Medicare nonparticipating fee schedule. This amount, 115 percent of the fee listed in the nonPAR MFS, is:

   A. Roster billing   C. Advance beneficiary notice
   B. Discounted fee for service   D. Limiting charge

4. The program designed to identify and address fraud, waste, and abuse is the:

   A. Recovery auditor program   C. Physician Quality Reporting
                                        System (PQRS)
   B. Medicare Integrity Program (MIP)   D. Medical Review (MR) Program

5. This pays for inpatient hospital care, skilled nursing facility care, home health care, and hospice care.

   A. Medicare Part A
   B. Medicare Part B
   C. Medicare Part C
   D. Medicare Part D

6. This helps beneficiaries pay for physician services, outpatient hospital services, medical equipment, and other supplies and services.

   A. Medicare Part A
   B. Medicare Part B
   C. Medicare Part C
   D. Medicare Part D

7. Authorized under the MMA, this provides voluntary Medicare prescription drug plans that are open to people who are eligible for Medicare.

   A. Medicare Part A
   B. Medicare Part B
   C. Medicare Part C
   D. Medicare Part D

8. Private insurance that beneficiaries may purchase to fill in some of the gaps or unpaid amounts in Medicare coverage.

   A. Medicare Advantage
   B. Medicare + Choice
   C. Medicare Part C
   D. Medigap insurance

9. An organization that is responsible for providing all Medicare-covered services, except for hospice care, in return for a predetermined capitated payment.

   A. Medicare Advantage
   B. Medicare Part B
   C. Medicare Part C
   D. Medigap insurance

10. Correspondence that details the services that patients were provided over a thirty-day period, the amounts charged, and the amounts they may be billed.

    A. Common Working File
    B. Medicare card
    C. Medical Review Program
    D. Medicare Summary Notice

SELF-QUIZ

1. Who manages Medicare?

2. Who is eligible for Medicare benefits?

3. What is a Medigap insurance policy?

4. What is Medicare's typical coinsurance?

5. What is covered by Medicare Part D?

CRITICAL THINKING QUESTIONS

1. What is the benefit of choosing Medicare Advantage rather than the Original Medicare Plan?

2. Why might a provider choose to accept assignment in some cases and not choose to accept assignment in other cases?

3. Why should individuals purchase Medigap insurance policies?

4. Is a disabled child eligible for Medicare benefits? If so, what HICN would be used?

5. Should persons who have the financial means to do so pay higher premiums or deductibles for the Medicare health care benefit?

WEB ACTIVITIES

SURFING THE NET

1. Go to the website of Medicare Part B—http://medicare.gov. Click on Medicare Basics, then click on Medicare Part B.
   A. What is the current deductible for Medicare Part B?

   _____

   _____

   B. What is the current coinsurance amount for Medicare Part B?

   _____

   _____

   C. What is the current premium for Medicare Part B?

   _____

   _____

2. Go to the website for Novitas Solutions, Inc., at: www.novitas-solutions.com/.
   A. In what capacity does this organization serve under Medicare Part A?

   _____

   _____

B. For whom is this website intended?

_____

_____

USING THE WEB WISELY

1. Using a search engine such as Yahoo or Google, locate a vendor of Medigap insurance in your area.

A. What types of plans are available?

_____

_____

B. Who is eligible to offer Medigap insurance in your state/area?

_____

_____

C. How can you tell if this is a reputable company?

_____

_____

WEB SCAVENGER HUNT

1. Go to the Social Security website, www.ssa.gov. Using the site's search feature:

A. How are social security numbers assigned?
B. How can you correct information on the social security card?
C. How can you receive a replacement card?
D. Are social security numbers reused?

APPLYING CONCEPTS

Part A

Mildred Johnson is a 67-year-old Medicare beneficiary. Her identification number is 235679010A. Today she is diagnosed with acquired hemolytic anemia (D59.9). Her physician suggested a B_{12} injection as treatment; however, he explained that Medicare will only pay for B_{12} injections for patients diagnosed with pernicious anemia (D51.0). The injection will cost $72; Mrs. Johnson has decided she will pay the cost if it is denied by Medicare.

Prepare a Medicare Advance Beneficiary Form for Mrs. Johnson's signature.

Part B

Students may wish to refer to the chapters on the introduction to the medical billing cycle and patient encounter and billing information in this workbook for a review of math for the following problems.

Dr. Augustino is a Medicare participating provider. Dr. Brunner is a Medicare nonparticipating provider who accepts assignment. Dr. Charles is a Medicare nonparticipating provider who does not accept assignment. The following table shows the fees each doctor charges as well as the Medicare Fee.

	Dr. A	Dr. B	Dr. C	Medicare
99201 OV New	45.00	42.50	48.00	36.00
99204 OV New	60.00	57.50	65.00	48.25
99212 OV Est	40.00	38.00	45.00	32.00
99213 OV Est	45.00	40.00	48.00	35.75
71020 Chest X-ray	165.00	162.50	174.00	73.25
36415 Venipuncture	17.00	12.00	20.00	8.00

- Audrey Appel, who is covered by Medicare as well as a Medigap policy, is a new patient of Dr. Augustino. She is seen in the office for an office visit, 99204, and has blood drawn for a lab test, 36415.

  1. For this patient, determine:

  (1) What amount Medicare pays the physician.
  (2) What amount the Medigap/supplemental plan pays.
  (3) What amount the patient pays.
  (4) What amount is written off.

- Benny Brown, who is covered by Medicare as well as a Medigap policy, is an established patient of Dr. Brunner. He comes to the office complaining of difficulty breathing. After a problem-focused examination and medical history, 99213, he also receives a chest X-ray, 71020.

  2. For this patient, determine:

  (1) What amount Medicare pays the physician.
  (2) What amount the Medigap/supplemental plan pays.
  (3) What amount the patient pays.
  (4) What amount is written off.

- Cathy Craine, who is covered by Medicare but does not have a Medigap policy, is a new patient of Dr. Charles. She is seen for a minor cold, 99201.

  3. For this patient, determine:

  (1) What amount Medicare pays the physician.
  (2) What amount the Medigap/supplemental plan pays.
  (3) What amount the patient pays.
  (4) What amount is written off.

Part C

The following was issued as a press release by BCBS of Illinois.

> **BlueCross BlueShield of Illinois offers Plans K and L**
>
> BlueCross BlueShield of Illinois announced two new low-cost, cost-sharing Medicare supplement plans for Illinois seniors, Plans K and L. These plans aim to help individuals seeking assistance with the portion of doctor and hospital bills that Medicare does not cover, Business Wire, Inc. reports.
>
> Plans K and L are options for seniors seeking lower premiums for their supplemental insurance. They provide coverage comparable to other Medicare supplement products but have lower monthly premiums in exchange for higher cost-sharing by the member.
>
> Members with Plan K pay half of the cost-sharing for covered services (such as the first-day deductible for hospital care). Members with Plan L pay 25 percent for these services. Once members reach an out-of-pocket limit ($4,000 for Plan K and $2,000 for Plan L), 100 percent of their Medicare copayments and coinsurances are covered for the rest of the calendar year.

- Yolanda Younes-Garcia of Decatur, IL, has decided to purchase BCBS Plan K. She has a $15 copay and 50-50 coinsurance. She has met $3,945 of her out-of-pocket expenses this year. Her physician charges $345 for an annual physical.

    (1) What amount will Yolanda pay?
    (2) What amount will Medicare pay?

If Yolanda is seen for a follow-up office visit after her annual physical:
    (3) What amount will she pay?
    (4) What amount will Medicare pay?

Medicaid

Chapter 10

Learning Outcomes

After studying this chapter, you should be able to:

10.1 Discuss the purpose of the Medicaid program.

10.2 Discuss general eligibility requirements for Medicaid.

10.3 Assess the income and asset guidelines used by most states to determine eligibility.

10.4 Evaluate the importance of verifying a patient's Medicaid enrollment.

10.5 Explain the services that Medicaid usually does not cover.

10.6 Describe the types of plans that states offer Medicaid recipients.

10.7 Discuss the claim filing procedures when a Medicaid recipient has other insurance coverage.

10.8 Prepare accurate Medicaid claims.

ASSISTED OUTLINING

Directions: *Read the chapter through one time. Then go back over the chapter and find the information required to complete the following outline of the chapter. Write the requested information directly in the spaces provided.*

1. How is Medicaid funded?

2. Who runs Medicaid?

10.1 The Medicaid Program

1. How and when was Medicaid established?

2. What is the purpose of Medicaid?

3. How is Medicaid funded?

4. How is Medicaid eligibility determined?

5. How does one apply for Medicaid?

6. Explain how Medicaid coverage works.

10.2 Eligibility

1. Explain categorically needy.

2. List five of the nine groups to which states extend benefits.

   (1)   (4)

   (2)   (5)

   (3)

3. What is meant by TANF?

Children's Health Insurance Program

4. Who is covered under CHIP?

5. How are the CHIP programs funded?

6. What is covered by CHIP programs?

7. How do states meet CHIP requirements?

Early and Periodic Screening, Diagnosis, and Treatment

8. Who is covered by EPSDT?

9. What is the emphasis of EPSDT programs?

10. What is covered under EPSDT?

The Ticket to Work and Work Incentives Improvement Act

11. Explain the TWWIIA.

New Freedom Initiative

12. What is the purpose of the New Freedom Initiative?

Spousal Impoverishment Protection

13. How does spousal impoverishment legislation protect spouses?

14. What specific assets are protected?

Welfare Reform Act

15. How has welfare reform changed eligibility for Medicaid?

16. Who determines eligibility for Temporary Assistance for Needy Families (TANF)?

17. What is considered when determining eligibility?

10.3 State Programs

1. How do states establish eligibility for Medicaid programs?

2. Explain medically needy.

3. Give five examples of groups covered by state rules but not federal guidelines.

(1)   (4)

(2)   (5)

(3)

Income and Asset Guidelines

4. What guidelines do most states use in determining eligibility?

Spend-Down Programs

5. How do spend-down programs work?

10.4 Medicaid Enrollment Verification

Insurance Procedures

1. How is a patient's Medicaid eligibility verified?

2. What is a restricted plan under Medicaid?

3. How is a Medicaid-eligible patient's identity verified?

Medicaid Fraud and Abuse

4. How can states increase their federal recovery amount?

5. What provisions must be included in the employee handbooks of large facilities such as hospitals that receive Medicaid payments of or exceeding $5 million?

10.5 Covered and Excluded Services

1. How are services and payment rates determined?

Covered Services

2. List services that states must cover to receive federal matching funds.

(1)   (5)

(2)   (6)

(3)   (7)

(4)   (8)

3. List three of the most common optional services that receive matching funds from the federal government.

(1)   (3)

(2)

Excluded Services

4. How are services not covered under Medicaid handled?

5. What are two of these types of services?

(1)   (2)

10.6 Plans and Payments

Fee-for-Service

1. How do fee-for-service plans work for Medicaid clients?

Managed Care

2. What is the current trend for coverage of Medicaid clients?

3. How do managed care plans work for Medicaid clients?

4. What are some of the advantages of managed care plans for Medicaid clients?

5. How are Medicaid managed care claims handled?

Payment for Services

6. How do providers become eligible to treat Medicaid patients?

7. How are providers paid for treating Medicaid clients?

8. What, if any, contribution does the Medicaid patient pay?

9. What services are exempt from copayments for Medicaid patients?

10. When can the patient be billed?

11. When is it not possible to bill the patient?

12. What is a utilization review?

10.7 Third-Party Liability

Payer of Last Resort

1. Explain the concept of payer of last resort for Medicaid.

Medicare-Medicaid Crossover Claims

2. What is meant by Medi-Medi beneficiaries? What is another term that means the same?

3. How are claims for Medi-Medi patients handled? What is the term used to identify these claims?

10.8 Claim Filing and Completion Guidelines

1. Who handles the claim filing guidelines for Medicaid?

Where to File

2. How do the states handle Medicaid claims submission?

Medicaid Coding

3. How is coding affected when filing Medicaid claims?

Fraudulent Billing Practices

4. List the four unacceptable Medicaid billing practices.

(1)   (3)

(2)   (4)

After Filing

5. How does the provider know the outcome once a claim has been submitted?

6. What are the steps in appealing a Medicaid claim that has been denied?

Medicaid Claim Completion

7. What formats may be used to submit Medicaid claims?

HIPAA Claims

8. When using the HIPAA 837P claim, what special data elements may be required by state guidelines?

9. How is the physician's Medicaid number reported on HIPAA 837P claims?

KEY TERMS
DEFINITIONS

Define the following terms:

1. Categorically needy

2. Dual-eligible

3. Early and Periodic Screening, Diagnosis, and Treatment (EPSDT)

4. Medically needy

5. Payer of last resort

6. Restricted status

7. Spend-down

8. Children's Health Insurance Program (CHIP)

9. Temporary Assistance for Needy Families (TANF)

10. Welfare Reform Act

SELF-QUIZ

1. Why do Medicaid plans vary from state to state?

2. How long may most recipients receive TANF payments?

3. What is the difference between categorically needy and medically needy?

4. Who determines coverage for Medicaid? What guidelines must be followed?

5. How can the medical billing specialist properly identify Medicaid recipients?

CRITICAL THINKING QUESTIONS

1. Why is it important to check both the patient's Medicaid card and another form of identification?

2. Why are states moving away from fee-for-service and toward managed care plans for Medicaid clients?

3. What are the sociological implications of CHIP programs?

4. Why doesn't the federal government run all Medicaid plans?

5. What are some positive and some negative reasons for a provider to participate in Medicaid?

WEB ACTIVITIES

SURFING THE NET

1. Using your favorite search engine or Table 10.1 in the textbook, locate the website of your state's Medicaid plan. (You may need to use search terms such as *Medicaid, medical assistance plan, public welfare, public assistance*, the plus symbol, and your state's name.)

A. Where/how do persons in your state apply for Medicaid benefits?

_____

_____

B. What are the eligibility requirements?

_____

_____

C. Does your state offer fee-for-service or managed care coverage, or both?

_____

_____

D. Are providers able to access information from this website?

_____

_____

(1) What type of information is available?

_____

_____

USING THE WEB WISELY

1. Using your favorite search engine, locate information, articles, position papers, etc., that give either positive or negative viewpoints on Medicaid programs.

A. What is the viewpoint of the writer?

_____

_____

(1) Does the writer have any specific political, religious, or other point of view?

_____

_____

B. What is the purpose of publishing this material?

_____

_____

C. How old is the information? How old is the date, if any is used, that supports the writers' viewpoint?

_____

_____

D. Do you agree or disagree with the writer?

_____

_____

APPLYING CONCEPTS

These patients are being seen by Dr. Christopher Connolly of Valley Associates, P.C. (Dr. Connolly's practice information is shown on page 487 in the textbook.)

1. A new patient is being seen today by Dr. Christopher Connolly. His name is Brian Kehoe, and he is insured by a Medicaid managed care plan. The doctor accepts assignment. His copay is $10, which he paid today. He is examined in the office today for an abscess on his mouth, which is not related to any type of accident.

   Encounter Form Data

Diagnosis 1	K12.2, abscess of mouth
Procedure Code	99201
Procedure Cost	$70

If Medicaid pays 50 percent of the physician's usual charge, after applying the copay, what payment will Medicaid send?

2. Karly Raub, an established patient of Dr. Connolly, was seen in our office today for ventricular fibrillation. She is currently unemployed and presents a current Medicaid card.

   Encounter Form Data

Diagnosis 1	I49.01, Ventricular fibrillation
Diagnosis 2	I10, Essential hypertension
Procedure Code	99212
Procedure Cost	$65
Procedure Code	93000, ECG Complete
Procedure Cost	$95

If Medicaid pays 45 percent of the physician's usual charge and applies the $10 that Karly paid today for her copay, what payment will Medicaid send?

TRICARE and CHAMPVA

Chapter 11

Learning Outcomes

After studying this chapter, you should be able to:

11.1 Discuss the eligibility requirements for TRICARE.
11.2 Compare TRICARE participating and nonparticipating providers.
11.3 Explain how the TRICARE Standard, TRICARE Prime, and TRICARE Extra programs differ.
11.4 Discuss the TRICARE for Life program.
11.5 Discuss the eligibility requirements for CHAMPVA.
11.6 Prepare accurate TRICARE and CHAMPVA claims.

ASSISTED OUTLINING

Directions: *Read the chapter through one time. Then go back over the chapter and find the information required to complete the following outline of the chapter. Write the requested information directly in the spaces provided.*

11.1 The TRICARE Program

1. What is TRICARE?

2. What was the name of the previous program?

3. What facilities are included in the TRICARE program?

4. Who is eligible for TRICARE?

5. What is the term used to designate the uniformed services member?

6. Who makes decisions about eligibility?

7. What should the medical billing specialist do when a TRICARE patient arrives for treatment?

8. Where is information about patient eligibility stored?

9. Who may contact DEERS?

11.2 Provider Participation and Nonparticipation

1. What is a TRICARE authorized provider?

Participating Providers

2. What is meant by a participating TRICARE provider?

Nonparticipating Providers

3. How is medical billing different for a nonparticipating TRICARE provider?

4. What is cost-share?

5. How is payment made for nonparticipating providers?

Reimbursement

6. How are participating providers paid by TRICARE?

Network and Non-network Providers

7. How are network and non-network providers paid?

11.3 TRICARE Plans

TRICARE Standard

1. What is TRICARE Standard?

2. What is covered under TRICARE Standard?

3. How are specific costs shared under TRICARE Standard?

4. What is a catastrophic cap?

Covered Services

5. List six services typically covered under TRICARE Standard.

(1)   (4)

(2)   (5)

(3)   (6)

Noncovered Services

6. List three services generally not covered by TRICARE Standard.

(1)   (3)

(2)

7. Where are individuals encouraged to first seek care under TRICARE Standard?

8. What is a NAS?

9. When must a NAS be obtained?

Preauthorization Requirements

10. Are outpatient NAS required? When?

11. List four outpatient procedures that normally require preauthorization.

(1)   (3)

(2)   (4)

TRICARE Prime

12. What is TRICARE Prime?

13. How is patient care managed?

14. How do non-active duty members become eligible for TRICARE Prime?

15. What are the deductibles and copays for TRICARE Prime?

TRICARE Prime Remote

16. What are the criteria to be eligible for TRICARE Prime Remote?

TRICARE Extra

17. What is TRICARE Extra?

18. What are the costs for TRICARE Extra?

TRICARE Reserve Select

19. What is TRICARE Reserve Select?

11.4 TRICARE and Other Insurance Plans

1. How does the medical billing specialist handle billing if the member also has other insurance?

2. What purpose would supplemental insurance policies serve for TRICARE beneficiaries?

TRICARE for Life

3. What is TRICARE for Life? How was it previously known?

4. What is the benefit of enrolling in TRICARE for Life?

5. When a beneficiary has TRICARE for Life and Medicare coverage, which is the primary payer?

11.5 CHAMPVA

1. What is CHAMPVA?

2. What is the effect of the Veterans Health Care Eligibility Reform Act of 1996?

Eligibility

3. Who determines eligibility for CHAMPVA?

4. Who is eligible for CHAMPVA benefits?

CHAMPVA Authorization Card

5. What is an A-Card? How is it used?

Covered Services

6. What services are covered by CHAMPVA?

7. List five inpatient and five outpatient services that are covered.

    (1) Inpatient services
        (a)
        (b)
        (c)
        (d)
        (e)

    (2) Outpatient services
        (a)
        (b)
        (c)
        (d)
        (e)

Excluded Services

8. List the four services that are usually not covered by CHAMPVA.

    (1)   (3)

    (2)   (4)

Preauthorization

9. Who is responsible for obtaining preauthorization?

10. List three procedures that require CHAMPVA preauthorization.

(1)   (3)

(2)

11. Do CHAMPVA enrollees need to obtain nonavailability statements? Why or why not?

Participating Providers

12. How are participating providers determined?

13. What are the payment ramifications of treating CHAMPVA patients?

Costs

14. What is the cost to the enrollee for CHAMPVA coverage?

15. How much is typical CHAMPVA reimbursement?

CHAMPVA and Other Health Insurance Plans

16. How does the medical billing specialist handle CHAMPVA when the patient has other health insurance?

CHAMPVA for Life

17. What is CHAMPVA for Life?

11.6 Filing Claims

1. How does the medical billing specialist handle TRICARE for Life claims?

2. When can an individual file claims?

HIPAA and TRICARE

3. How is TRICARE affected by HIPAA?

Fraud and Abuse

4. Who oversees concerns about fraud and abuse in TRICARE programs?

5. Are other reviews used with TRICARE programs?

6. If fraud or abuse is determined, what are the possible penalties?

Filing CHAMPVA Claims

7. How are CHAMPVA for Life claims filed?

KEY TERMS

MATCHING

Match the definition with the correct term from the following word list.

A. catastrophic cap	I. TRICARE
B. CHAMPUS	J. TRICARE Extra
C. CHAMPVA	K. TRICARE for Life
D. cost-share	L. TRICARE Prime
E. DEERS	M. TRICARE Prime Remote
F. Military Treatment Facility (MTF)	N. TRICARE Standard
G. nonavailability statement (NAS)	O. TRICARE Reserve Select
H. Primary Care Manager (PCM)	

1. The previous name for TRICARE.

2. A program for purchase by certain members of the National Guard and Reserve called up after September 11, 2001.

3. This is who is contacted with questions regarding eligibility.

4. An electronic document stating that the service the patient requires is not available at the nearby military treatment facility.

5. A managed care plan under TRICARE for persons wishing to receive services primarily from civilian facilities.

6. A program for Medicare-eligible military retirees and Medicare-eligible family members.

7. Enrollees in this program receive the majority of their health care services from military treatment facilities and receive priority at these facilities.

8. The government's health insurance program for veterans with a 100 percent service-related disability and their families.

9. A fee-for-service program that replaces the CHAMPUS program.

10. A limit on the total medical expenses that beneficiaries are required to pay in one year.

SELF-QUIZ

1. What is the main difference between TRICARE Standard and TRICARE Prime? What is the main difference between TRICARE Prime and TRICARE Prime Remote?

2. Can the medical billing specialist contact DEERS? Why or why not?

3. Who is eligible for CHAMPVA benefits?

4. What is an A-card? How is it used by the medical billing specialist?

5. What is a nonavailability statement?

CRITICAL THINKING QUESTIONS

1. Why might a retired military person prefer to keep TRICARE for Life rather than enroll in Medicare?

2. Is the surgeon general covered by TRICARE benefits? Why or why not?

3. Why should active-duty military personnel be able to receive care at non-military facilities?

4. Why would a person choose TRICARE Extra over TRICARE Standard?

5. Why do you think CHAMPUS was replaced with TRICARE?

WEB ACTIVITIES

SURFING THE NET

1. Go to TRICARE's website, www.tricare.mil.

    A. Using the link TRICARE Regions (or the map), click on your region.

    _____

    _____

    B. At the screen dedicated to the region in which you live, click on Find a Provider.

    _____

    _____

C. Locate providers in your city for persons covered by TRICARE Prime.

_____

_____

D. Locate providers in your city for persons covered by TRICARE Standard.
   (1) From your search results, do any of the providers accept both TRICARE Prime and TRICARE Standard patients?

_____

_____

WEB SCAVENGER HUNT

1. Go to TRICARE's Fraud and Abuse website, www.tricare.mil/fraud.

   A. Click on the Reporting Fraud link.
   B. Who should be contacted in your geographic area to report fraud?
   C. Who should be contacted to report pharmacy fraud?

2. Return to the TRICARE Fraud and Abuse home page.

   A. Click on the Sanctions link.
   B. Using the search screen that comes up, select the abbreviation for your state. (If you get zero results, select a neighboring state.)
   C. How many providers have been sanctioned?
   D. What are the reasons for the providers being sanctioned?
   E. Have any providers lost their license to practice medicine?

APPLYING CONCEPTS

Students may wish to refer to the chapters on the introduction to the medical billing cycle and patient encounter and billing information in this workbook for a review of math for the following problems.

1. Pete Weiskner is a retired Air Force captain; he is covered by TRICARE Standard. He recently had an annual colonoscopy as he has a family history of colon cancer. The procedure was performed by a nonparticipating provider. The total allowed charge was $832; the provider billed Pete $956.80. Pete has met his annual deductible.

   (1) What amount will Pete be responsible for?

   (2) What amount will be reimbursed by TRICARE?

2. Eva Logorda's husband Angelo is completely disabled due to a service-related injury. When Eva comes to your office, you verify her eligibility through her A-card. She notes that she has a $100 deductible and has met $49 of the deductible for this year. Today she receives a complete physical exam; the charges total $276.

   (1) What amount will Eva be responsible for?

   (2) What amount will be reimbursed by CHAMPVA?

3. Leon Rosen recently retired from the Navy. He and his wife, Miriam, must choose a TRICARE health plan. They have decided to use a typical office visit, with total charges of $45, as an example to help determine the best plan for them. Assume they have met any deductible, premiums, or other fees to enroll in the program.

(1) What is the out-of-pocket amount for the office visit under TRICARE Standard?

(2) What is the out-of-pocket amount for the office visit under TRICARE Prime?

(3) What is the out-of-pocket amount for the office visit under TRICARE Extra?

Chapter 12 Workers' Compensation and Disability/Automotive Insurance

Learning Outcomes

After studying this chapter, you should be able to:

12.1 Explain the four federal workers' compensation plans.
12.2 Describe the two types of state workers' compensation benefits
12.3 Classify work-related injuries.
12.4 List three responsibilities of the physician of record in a workers' compensation case.
12.5 Differentiate between Social Security Disability Insurance (SSDI) and Supplemental Security Income (SSI).

ASSISTED OUTLINING

Directions: *Read the chapter through one time. Then go back over the chapter and find the information required to complete the following outline of the chapter. Write the requested information directly in the spaces provided.*

1. Before OSHA, how could injured workers receive compensation for their injuries?

2. How and when was OSHA created?

3. What is the purpose of OSHA?

4. What happens if businesses do not meet OSHA standards?

5. Who is exempt from OSHA legislation?

6. What can an employee do if he or she believes the work environment is unhealthy or unsafe?

7. May the employee suffer negative consequences for filing an OSHA complaint?

12.1 Federal Workers' Compensation Plans

1. How are civilian federal workers covered?

2. Who oversees the Office of Workers' Compensation Programs (OWCP)?

3. List and explain the four programs under the OWCP.

(1)   (3)

(2)   (4)

4. What is provided by each of these programs for ill or injured workers?

12.2 State Workers' Compensation Plans

1. What two types of workers' compensation must all states provide?

2. List three sources of workers' compensation insurance.

(1)   (3)

(2)

3. How does a state workers' compensation fund operate?

4. What are the benefits of using private insurance carriers?

5. What is meant by self-insured?

6. Who pays for workers' compensation?

7. How can states and workers verify that an employer carries workers' compensation insurance?

Eligibility

8. Who is eligible for coverage by a workers' compensation policy?

9. What happens to companies that fail to carry workers' compensation insurance?

10. List six categories of employers who are generally NOT required to carry workers' compensation insurance.

(1)   (4)

(2)   (5)

(3)   (6)

Benefits

11. What is covered by workers' compensation insurance?

12. Must the employee be injured on the premises of the business to collect benefits?

13. Explain what an occupational disease or illness is.

14. How are medical benefits paid by most states?

15. What are typical methods of determining wage-loss benefits?

16. What benefits are available to the family of a worker killed on the job?

Covered Injuries and Illnesses

17. Who determines what injuries are covered under workers' compensation?

18. What four criteria must an injury generally meet to be covered by workers' compensation?

    (1)   (3)

    (2)   (4)

19. What are two types of accidents? Give an example of each.

20. List four types of injuries that are generally covered by state programs.

    (1)   (3)

    (2)   (4)

21. List four conditions that can cause injuries to be excluded from workers' compensation.

    (1)   (3)

    (2)   (4)

12.3 Workers' Compensation Terminology

Classification of Injuries

1. What are the five categories of work-related injuries?

    (1)   (4)

    (2)   (5)

    (3)

Injury without Disability

2. Explain injury without disability.

Injury with Temporary Disability

3. Explain injury with temporary disability.

Injury with Permanent Disability

4. Explain injury with permanent disability.

5. What is an independent medical examination?

6. How are expenses and lost wages paid for a worker with a permanent disability?

7. How is the amount of compensation determined?

Injury Requiring Vocational Rehabilitation

8. Explain injury requiring vocational rehabilitation.

9. What is vocational rehabilitation?

Injury Resulting in Death

10. Explain injury resulting in death.

Pain and Disability

11. How do physicians describe the illnesses or injuries under workers' compensation?

Pain Terminology

12. What are the four classifications of pain?

(1)   (3)

(2)   (4)

Disability Terminology

13. List and explain the six ways disabilities due to spinal injuries, heart disease, pulmonary disease, or abdominal weakness are classified.

(1)   (4)

(2)   (5)

(3)   (6)

14. What are the two descriptions of disabilities to the lower extremities?

(1)   (2)

Workers' Compensation and the HIPAA Privacy Rule

15. How is privacy for workers' compensation cases affected by HIPAA?

16. List three instances when access to workers' compensation files is unrestricted by HIPAA.

(1)   (3)

(2)

17. How does this affect disclosure of information about the workers' previous condition?

12.4 Claim Process

1. List the steps in the claim process.

Responsibilities of the Physician of Record

2. Define physician of record.

3. What are the responsibilities of the physician of record?

4. How are providers paid?

5. What types of codes must be included to report the cause of the accident?

Responsibilities of the Employer and Insurance Carrier

6. What is in the first report of injury form?

7. Who files the first report of injury and when is it filed?

8. What steps are taken by the insurance carrier?

9. What is the difference between an admission of liability and a notice of contest?

10. How is the employee compensated?

11. If the claim is denied, what is the employee's responsibility?

Termination of Compensation and Benefits

12. List four of the seven reasons for temporary partial or temporary total disability benefits to end.

(1)   (3)

(2)   (4)

Appeals

13. What is the appeal process?

Billing and Claim Management

14. What is the importance of the first medical treatment report?

15. How should information related to an established patient be recorded for a workers' compensation claim?

16. When an established patient makes an appointment for an injury that may have occurred on the job, what questions should the scheduler ask?

17. If the case is a workers' compensation claim, what steps must the medical billing specialist take prior to the first appointment?

18. What claim forms may be used for workers' compensation claims?

19. What are some general guidelines for completing claims?

12.5 Disability Compensation and Automotive Insurance Programs

1. What do disability compensation programs cover? Not cover?

2. How can an individual receive compensation under a disability program?

Private Programs

3. How do employees receive/purchase disability insurance?

Government Programs

4. List the five major government disability benefit programs.

   (1)   (4)

   (2)   (5)

   (3)

Social Security Disability Insurance (SSDI)

5. How is SSDI funded?

6. What benefit does SSDI provide?

7. What federal act allows for payroll deduction for SSDI coverage?

8. How is disability defined by SSDI in Section 223(d) of the Social Security Act?

9. What three categories of disability are eligible for coverage under SSDI?

   (1)   (3)

   (2)

10. Who is eligible for disability benefits under SSDI?

11. How long does the SSDI application process take?

12. When can individuals receiving SSDI apply for additional Medicare disability benefits?

Supplemental Security Income (SSI)

13. What benefits does SSI provide?

14. How is SSI different from SSDI?

15. Who is eligible for SSI benefits?

16. What is the SSI basic benefit?

Federal Worker Disability Programs

17. How are federal workers covered for disability?

18. What are the components of the FERS program?

19. How do FERS and SSDI benefits work together?

20. What are the disability criteria of CSRS? How do they compare with SSDI?

21. How does a worker qualify for disability?

22. How may federal employees receive health care benefits when disabled?

Veterans Programs

23. What two programs cover veterans?

   (1)   (2)

24. Who is eligible for coverage under the Veterans Compensation Program?

25. Who is eligible for coverage under the Veterans Pension Program?

Preparing Disability Reports

26. How are disability reports created?

27. What medical information should be included in the disability report?

28. List two ways the provider may bill for time spent preparing disability reports.

   (1)   (2)

Automobile Insurance

29. What is an automobile insurance policy?

30. Explain personal injury protection (PIP).

31. What are liens?

Subrogation

32. Describe subrogation as it relates to workers' compensation or liability/automotive claims.

KEY TERMS

MULTIPLE CHOICE

Circle the letter of the choice that best matches the definition or answers the question.

1. A welfare program that provides financial assistance to individuals in need, including aged, blind, and disabled individuals.

   A. SSDI   **C.** SSI
   B. OWCP   **D.** OSHA

2. A federal program that provides compensation for lost wages due to disability.

   A. SSDI   **C.** SSI
   B. OWCP   **D.** OSHA

3. Employee payroll deductions that are used to partially fund Social Security Disability Insurance (SSDI).

   A. SSDI   **C.** SSI
   B. FECA   **D.** FICA

4. What report is filed by the physician in state workers' compensation cases when a patient's medical condition or disability changes?

   A. First report   **C.** Progress report
   B. First report of injury   **D.** Notice of Contest

5. This organization seeks to protect workers from health and safety risks on the job.

   A. SSDI   **C.** SSI
   B. OWCP   **D.** OSHA

6. Conditions that develop as a result of workplace conditions or activities.

   A. Layoffs   **C.** Occupational diseases or illnesses
   B. Progress reports   **D.** Vocational rehabilitation

7. The form, usually filed within 24 hours of injury or illness, that contains information about the patient, the employer, and the injury or illness.

   A. Final report   **C.** Physician of record
   B. First report of injury   **D.** Notice of Contest

8. The act provides workers' compensation benefits to individuals employed by the federal government.

   A. OWCP   **C.** FECA
   B. FICA   **D.** OSHA

9. The physician who first treats the injured or ill employee is known as the:

   A. Final report
   B. Final report of injury
   C. Progress report
   D. Physician of record

10. A determination that the employer is not liable for the worker's injury or illness.

   A. Notice of Contest
   B. First Report of Injury
   C. Admission of Liability
   D. Final report

SELF-QUIZ

1. Who purchases and/or pays for workers' compensation insurance?

2. How are federal workers covered by workers' compensation insurance?

3. Who is eligible for SSDI?

4. Who is eligible for SSI?

5. What medical information should be included in the disability report?

CRITICAL THINKING QUESTIONS

1. What is the difference between SSI and SSDI?

2. Why should a person purchase disability insurance?

3. Why is it important to not take a job that pays "under the table"?

4. Why should a separate medical record/chart be created for an established patient being seen for an occupational illness or injury?

5. Should people who qualify for SSI or SSDI be re-evaluated for eligibility as time passes?

WEB ACTIVITIES

USING THE WEB WISELY

1. Using a search engine such as Google or Yahoo, search for companies that sell disability insurance to individuals. Locate two companies.

   A. Using the company websites, what types of benefits are paid by disability insurance?

   _____

   _____

   B. If possible, obtain a quote for purchasing a disability insurance policy from each company. Compare the prices between the two companies.

   _____

   _____

2. Can you determine who the parent company of the disability insurance company is? (In some instances, there is no parent company.)

   _____

   _____

   A. What is the reputation of each of these companies?

   _____

   _____

WEB SCAVENGER HUNT

1. Search for the website for workers' compensation in your state.
   A. Locate the entry for the department, division, bureau, etc., for workers' compensation and click on the link. (Each state uses different terminology to identify the portion of state government that deals with workers' compensation.)
      (1) Can you find a printable First Report of Injury form on this website? (Many states now have online filing of First Report of Injury forms; however, often you can still locate a link to print a paper copy.)
   B. Next, find the website for another state's workers' compensation program.
      (1) Locate the First Report of Injury form on this website.
      (2) Compare the forms of the two states. How are they alike? Different?

2. Sample electronic forms are available by going to www.interfacetec.com.
   A. At the Interface Technologies website, click on Demo Download Center, then scroll to the listing of workers' compensation forms.
      (1) Can you locate a sample form for First Report of Injury?
      (2) What is the purpose of this website?

APPLYING CONCEPTS

1. Using the information in Case 12.1 on pages 421–422 of the textbook plus the additional information given below, complete the Ohio Workers' Compensation Commission's First Report of Injury form for Mr. Puopolo. A blank form is located at the back of the workbook.

Injured worker information

Dependents: 3

Department name: Repair Department

Wage rate: $17.78 hour

Work schedule: Monday through Friday, 8 a.m. to 4 p.m.

Job title: Senior mechanic

Wages and payment: None expected from other than Ohio Bureau of Workers' Compensation

Treatment information

Employer address: 4829 West Main Street, Toledo, OH 43602-0979

Place of accident: Property of JV Trucking

Date of accident: June 2, 2016

Time of accident: 10:50 a.m.

Date returned to work:

Date hired: April 13, 1998

State where hired: Ohio

Date employer notified: June 2, 2016

Description of accident: In Mr. Puopolo's exact words, "I was working on the front driver's side wheel when it came loose off the axle and fell on my right leg. It pinned my leg against the fender and I heard and felt a crack."

Type of injury/disease: Broken right leg

Number of work days missed: 3 days

Injury causally related to the industrial accident: yes

11-digit BWC provider number: 26875943158

Date of provider's signature: June 5, 2016

Employer information

Employer policy number: 569QH15736

Employer telephone: 555-322-4662

Federal ID number: 21-2697854

Emergency room treatment: yes

Hospitalized overnight: yes

Treatment away from work site: Valley Associates, P.C. and
Toledo Hospital
2142 North Cove Road
Toledo, OH 43606

Payments (RAs), Appeals, and Secondary Claims

Learning Outcomes

After studying this chapter, you should be able to:

13.1 Explain the claim adjudication process.

13.2 Describe the procedures for following up on claims after they are sent to payers.

13.3 Interpret a remittance advice (RA).

13.4 Identify the points that are reviewed on an RA.

13.5 Explain the process for posting payments and managing denials.

13.6 Describe the purpose and general steps of the appeal process.

13.7 Assess how appeals, postpayment audits, and overpayments may affect claim payments.

13.8 Describe the procedures for filing secondary claims.

13.9 Discuss procedures for complying with the Medicare Secondary Payer (MSP) program.

ASSISTED OUTLINING

Directions: Read the chapter through one time. Then go back over the chapter and find the information required to complete the following outline of the chapter. Write the requested information directly in the spaces provided.

1. What is the purpose of claim follow-up and payment processing?

13.1 Claim Adjudication

1. What is the first step made by the payer when processing a claim?

2. What is adjudication? What five steps are involved?

    (1)   (4)

    (2)   (5)

    (3)

Initial Processing

3. How are paper claims or paper attachments handled by the payer?

4. What happens when there is an error on a claim?

5. What should the medical billing specialist do when a claim is rejected?

Automated Review

6. What is an automated review?

7. What ten items are checked in the automated review?

(1)	(6)
(2)	(7)
(3)	(8)
(4)	(9)
(5)	(10)

8. What is concurrent care?

9. What process is followed when concurrent care is reported?

Manual Review

10. What happens if a problem is found in the automated review?

11. What is meant by development?

12. What is the process for claims in development?

13. What is the importance of documentation in the claim development process?

14. How is medical necessity typically decided in the claim review?

Determination

15. What is determination?

16. What is a medical necessity denial?

Payment

17. Explain the purpose of the RA/ERA.

18. What is an EOB?

19. How is payment typically handled?

13.2 Monitoring Claim Status

1. Define accounts receivable.

2. Who owes the monies known as A/R?

Claim Status

3. What two types of information are needed to monitor claims?

(1)   (2)

Claim Turnaround Time

4. What is meant by claim turnaround time?

5. What is a prompt-pay law?

Aging

6. What is aging?

7. What is the purpose of an insurance aging report?

HIPAA Health Care Claim Status Inquiry/Response

8. When do most practices begin the follow-up procedure for claims?

9. What is the correct HIPAA electronic transaction used to check status of claims? The response to the inquiry?

10. List and define the five claim status category codes used in the HIPAA 277 transaction for the main types of responses.

(1)   (4)

(2)   (5)

(3)

Working with Payers

11. List three important claims processing procedures every medical billing specialist must know to get claims processed as quickly as possible.

(1)   (3)

(2)

12. How should the medical billing specialist handle miscalculated payments or failure to pay a claim on time?

13.3 The Remittance Advice (RA)

1. What is the purpose of the RA?

2. How are electronic versus paper RAs different?

Content of RAs

3. Describe the content of RAs.

4. What are the four major sections of the RAs?

   (1)   (3)

   (2)   (4)

Header Information

5. What is contained in the header information section of the RA?

Claim Information

6. What is contained, for each claim, in the claim information section of the RA?

7. List and explain the sixteen column headings used on the RA.

   (1)   (9)

   (2)   (10)

   (3)   (11)

   (4)   (12)

   (5)   (13)

   (6)   (14)

   (7)   (15)

   (8)   (16)

Totals

8. What is contained in the totals section of the RA?

Glossary

9. What is contained in the glossary section of the RA?

Adjustments

10. What does an adjustment indicate on the RA?

11. What four actions may the payer take when making an adjustment?

    (1)   (3)

    (2)   (4)

12. What are the three types of codes used to explain the adjustment?

    (1)   (3)

    (2)

13. Where do these codes originate?

Claims Adjustment Group Codes

14. List and explain the five claim adjustment group codes.

    (1)   (4)

    (2)   (5)

    (3)

Claim Adjustment Reason Codes

15. Why do payers use claim adjustment reason codes?

Remittance Advice Remark Codes

16. Define the abbreviation RAR.

17. What do the remittance advice remark codes provide?

18. Who maintains these codes? Who may use these codes?

19. What is the difference between M codes and N codes?

13.4 Reviewing RAs

1. How is the claim control number used?

2. How is each claim processed?

3. List the six steps used to double-check the remittance data.

    (1)   (4)

    (2)   (5)

    (3)   (6)

13.5 Procedures for Posting

1. Define EFT.

2. What regulations are to be mandated under the Affordable Care Act (ACA) as of January 1, 2014?

3. How are claims paid without using an EFT?

Posting and Applying Payments and Adjustments

4. What five key elements should be entered into the PMP?

(1)   (4)

(2)   (5)

(3)

5. How does autoposting work?

Reconciling Payments

6. Define reconciling.

Denial Management

7. When claims are denied, what are three typical problems and their solutions?

(1)   (3)

(2)

8. How can the medical billing specialist improve the rate of paid claims?

13.6 Appeals

1. What are some of the reasons that may change the amount of payment on a claim?

The General Appeal Process

2. What is an appeal?

3. Who may appeal?

4. Can you differentiate between claimant and appellant?

Basic Steps

5. What are the basic steps in handling appeals?

Options After Appeal Rejection

6. Who reviews appeals that payers reject?

7. What materials are needed to appeal after a rejection?

Medicare Appeals

8. How can denial for minor errors or omissions be reversed?

9. What legislation regulates the Medicare appeals process?

10. What is redetermination?

11. List the five steps in the Medicare appeals process.

(1)   (4)

(2)   (5)

(3)

13.7 Postpayment Audits, Refunds, and Grievances

Postpayment Audits

1. What are the purposes of postpayment audits? How is this accomplished?

Refunds of Overpayments

2. What is another term for overpayment?

3. What is an overpayment?

4. How are overpayments reimbursed?

5. List two reasons why a refund request may be challenged.

(1)   (2)

Overpayment Enforcement under FERA

6. What do the new provisions of the Fraud Enforcement and Recovery Act of 2009 (FERA) say?

Grievances

7. What is the purpose of filing a grievance?

8. What is the typical grievance process? Who handles grievances?

13.8 Billing Secondary Payers

1. What is the key item a secondary payer needs to know?

Electronic Claims

2. Where does the medical billing specialist get the information to create a claim for a secondary payer?

3. What is included with the claim to the secondary payer?

4. How does COB work with the secondary payer?

5. Does the medical billing specialist always submit claims to the secondary payer? Why or why not?

6. What is the typical message included when the primary payer forwards the COB transaction?

Paper Claims

7. How are paper claims for secondary payers handled?

13.9 The Medicare Secondary Payer (MSP) Program, Claims, and Payments

1. How is the Medicare Secondary Payer Program run?

2. What effect do HIPAA rules have on Medicare as a secondary payer?

Following MSP Rules

Over Age Sixty-Five and Employed

3. What are the criteria for Medicare to be the secondary payer for an individual over age 65?

4. List five instances when Medicare is always the primary payer.

(1)   (4)

(2)   (5)

(3)

Disabled

5. How is Medicare coverage for individuals under age 65 and disabled handled?

End-Stage Renal Disease (ESRD)

6. What is the relationship between COB and ESRD-based Medicare coverage?

Workers' Compensation

7. What is the priority of Medicare coverage for work-related injuries or illnesses?

8. How is coverage under the Federal Black Lung Program and Medicare handled?

Automobile, No-Fault, and Liability Insurance

9. For accident-related claims, how is Medicare handled?

Veterans' Benefits

10. What are the choices for veterans entitled to Medicare benefits?

Insurance Type Code

11. When is the insurance type code used? When is it not used?

MSP Claims and Payments

12. Must a claim be filed with Medicare if Medicare is the secondary payer?

13. Under MSP, what amount of the patient's coinsurance will Medicare pay?

14. What is used in calculating the three formulas for determining coinsurance payments for MSP patients?

15. If a patient's Medicare Part B deductible has been met, how much of the patient's coinsurance will Medicare pay as a secondary payer?

16. List and describe the three formulas for determining coinsurance payments for MSP patients.

(1)   (3)

(2)

17. How does Medicare determine the amount of payment?

TRICARE CMS-1500 Secondary Claims

18. List the six items on a paper claim that are filled in differently when TRICARE is the secondary payer.

(1)   (4)

(2)   (5)

(3)   (6)

Medicare and Medicaid

19. If a patient is covered by both Medicare and Medicaid (a Medi-Medi beneficiary), which is primary?

KEY TERMS

MATCHING

Match the definition with the correct term from the following word list.

A. Accounts receivable (A/R)	N. Explanation of benefits (EOB)
B. Adjustment	O. Grievance
C. Aging	P. Insurance aging report
D. Appeal	Q. Medicare Redetermination Notice (MRN)
E. Autoposting	R. Medicare Secondary Payer (MSP)
F. Claim adjustment group code	S. Overpayments
G. Claim adjustment reason code (CARC)	T. Pending
H. Claim status code	U. Reconciliation
I. Claimant	V. Redetermination
J. Claim turnaround time	W. Remittance advice (RA)
K. Determination	X. Remittance advice remark code (RARC)
L. Development	Y. Suspended
M. Electronic funds transfer (EFT)	

1. The person filing the appeal.

2. A transaction that explains the payment decisions to the provider.

3. An older term that now usually refers to the paper document that explains the payment decisions.

4. The term used by payers to indicate that more information is needed for claim processing.

5. Processing clean claims within a specified period of time, usually 30 to 60 days from the time of claim submission.

6. The period of time a payer has had the claim.

7. A claim review by an employee of the Medicare carrier who was not involved in the initial claim determination.

8. Payers use these codes to provide details about an adjustment.

9. Claim status during adjudication when the payer is developing the claim.

10. A report that lists the claims transmitted on each day and how long they have been in process with the payer.

11. From the payer's point of view, improper or excessive payments resulting from billing errors for which the provider owes refunds.

12. A decision whether to (1) pay it, (2) deny it, or (3) pay it at a reduced level.

SELF-QUIZ

1. What is an EFT?

2. When can Medicare be a secondary payer?

3. What are the five steps in the Medicare appeals process?

4. List and describe the three formulas for determining coinsurance payments for MSP patients.

5. What are the five steps in the adjudication process?

CRITICAL THINKING QUESTIONS

1. What is the difference between a RA and an EOB?

2. Why should the billing and claims departments have effective communication?

3. How can persons under age 65 be eligible for Medicare?

4. Why might payers set a minimum amount that must be involved in an appeal process?

5. What is the importance of the insurance aging report?

WEB ACTIVITIES

SURFING THE NET

1. Using a search engine such as Google or Yahoo, search for your state's insurance commission/department.

   A. Using the website, locate information on your state's prompt payment law.

   1. What is the payment time frame?

   _____

   _____

   2. What, if any, are the penalties for late payments?

   _____

   _____

WEB SCAVENGER HUNT

1. Go to the website for updates to claim adjustment reason codes and remark codes at www.wpc-edi.com/codes.
   A. Click on claim adjustment reason codes.
      1. When were these codes last updated?
      2. Explain claim adjustment reason code 27.
   B. Click on remittance advice remark codes.
      1. When were these codes last updated?
      2. Explain remittance advice remark code N356.
   C. Click on claim status codes.
      1. When were these codes last updated?
      2. How many codes are available for use under this heading?
      3. Explain claim status code 30.

APPLYING CONCEPTS

Students may wish to refer to the chapters on the introduction to the medical billing cycle and patient encounter and billing information in this workbook for a review of math for the following problems.

Joseph D'Amico is covered by BlueCross and Medicare. His BlueCross plan has an 85-15 coinsurance and a $100 deductible. This year's Medicare deductible is $110. He was seen in our office on January 11; charges for the office visit were $135. Claims were submitted to BlueCross as primary payer and to Medicare as secondary payer.

1. What amount will BlueCross be responsible for?

2. What amount will Medicare be responsible for?

3. What amount will Joseph be responsible for?

Joseph saw the doctor again in February. Charges for the office visit and tests were $215.

4. What amount will BlueCross be responsible for?

5. What amount will Medicare be responsible for?

6. What amount will Joseph be responsible for?

The RA on page 176 was received by your practice on February 26. Use it to complete the ledger card for Gloria B. Ramirez. (There may be extra lines on the ledger card.)

Patient ID	Patient Name	Plan	Date of Service	Pro-cedure	Provider Charge	Allowed Amount	Patient Payment (Coinsurance and Deductible)	Claim Adjust-ment Reason Code	PROV PAY
537-88-5267	Ramirez, Gloria B.	R-1	02/13–02/13	99214	$105.60	$59.00	$8.85	2	$50.15
348-99-2537	Finucula, Betty R.	R-1	01/15–01/15	99292	$88.00	$50.00	$7.50	2	$42.50
537-88-5267	Ramirez, Gloria B.	R-1	02/14–02/14	90732	$38.00	0	$38.00	49	0
760-57-5372	Jugal, Kurt T.	R-1	02/16–02/16	93975 99204	$580.00 $178.00	$261.00 $103.00	$139.15 $15.45	1 2	$121.85 $87.55
875-17-0098	Quan, Mary K.	PPO-3	02/16–02/16	20004	$192.00	$156.00	$31.20	2	$124.80
								TOTAL	$426.85

Gloria B. Ramirez
921 East Broad Street
Bethlehem, PA 18018
610-555-6012

Universal Health
ID #537-88-5267

Date/Pro		Charge	Payment/Adj	Balance
2/13	OV	105.60		105.60
2/14	IMU	38.00		38.00

7. What are Gloria's coinsurance percentages?

8. Why did Gloria's insurance pay only $50.15 rather than $59.00 toward the office visit?

9. Why didn't Gloria's insurance pay for the pneumonia vaccination?

Jody Ehninger is seen in Dr. Ramic's office for a routine diabetic checkup; the doctor also decides to complete some laboratory tests. Jody is insured by Metropolitan Insurance and has a $100 deductible and a 70-30 coinsurance. Dr. Ramic is a participating provider.

The following RA is received on March 1.

Dzanan Ramic, MD
1529 Cedar Street
Allentown, PA 18104

Patient: Jody Ehninger
Claim: 19087756345
ID: 098765432
Plan code: P-PAR
Med. Rec. No.: 04–JEHN8791

Proc Code	From Date	Thru Date	Treat-ment	Status Code	Amount Chrgd	Amount Allwd	Copay/ Deduct	Coins	Amount Apprvd	Patient Balance
99213	02/18	02/18	1	1	167.00	84.00	84.00	0.00	0.00	0.00
81000	02/18	02/18	1	1	19.25	11.00	11.00	0.00	0.00	0.00
80061	02/18	02/18	1	1,2	261.50	171.00	5.00	116.20	116.20	49.80
84152	02/18	02/18	1	10	189.00	0.00	0.00	0.00	0.00	0.00
90471 /90658	02/18	02/18	1	2	13.00	9.50	0.00	6.65	6.65	2.85
				Claim Totals	649.75	275.50	100.00	122.85	122.85	52.65

10. Explain the claim adjustment reason codes for each procedure.

11. Why is the payer not responsible for coinsurance for procedure codes 99213 and 81000?

12. What amounts are written off for this visit? Why?

After receiving a statement and paying her bill in March, Jody visits the doctor again on May 12; the doctor's fees and the payer's allowed amounts have changed. The charges are for an office visit, 99213, amount charged $172, amount allowed $86; and a urinalysis, 81000, amount charged $20.50, amount allowed $12.75.

13. What is the amount of coinsurance for this visit?

14. What is the amount of write-off for this visit?

15. Complete a ledger card for Jody Ehninger. The RA was received on May 20 and Jody paid on May 29.

<table>
<tr><td colspan="2">Jody Ehninger
23 Lark Lane
Allentown, PA 18104
610-555-1516</td><td colspan="2">Metropolitan
ID #098765432
Chart #04-JEHN8791</td></tr>
<tr><th>Date/Pro</th><th>Charge</th><th>Payment/Adj</th><th>Balance</th></tr>
<tr><td></td><td></td><td></td><td></td></tr>
<tr><td></td><td></td><td></td><td></td></tr>
<tr><td></td><td></td><td></td><td></td></tr>
<tr><td></td><td></td><td></td><td></td></tr>
<tr><td></td><td></td><td></td><td></td></tr>
<tr><td></td><td></td><td></td><td></td></tr>
<tr><td></td><td></td><td></td><td></td></tr>
<tr><td></td><td></td><td></td><td></td></tr>
<tr><td></td><td></td><td></td><td></td></tr>
<tr><td></td><td></td><td></td><td></td></tr>
<tr><td></td><td></td><td></td><td></td></tr>
<tr><td></td><td></td><td></td><td></td></tr>
<tr><td></td><td></td><td></td><td></td></tr>
<tr><td></td><td></td><td></td><td></td></tr>
<tr><td></td><td></td><td></td><td></td></tr>
</table>

Chapter 14 Patient Billing and Collections

Learning Outcomes

After studying this chapter, you should be able to:

14.1 Explain the structure of a typical financial policy.

14.2 Describe the purpose and content of patients' statements and the procedures for working with them.

14.3 Compare individual patient billing and guarantor billing.

14.4 Classify the responsibilities for each position that is typically part of billing and collections.

14.5 Describe the processes and methods used to collect outstanding balances.

14.6 Name the two federal laws that govern credit arrangements.

14.7 Discuss the tools that can be used to locate unresponsive or missing patients.

14.8 Describe the procedures for clearing uncollectible balances.

14.9 Analyze the purpose of a retention schedule.

ASSISTED OUTLINING

Directions: Read the chapter through one time. Then go back over the chapter and find the information required to complete the following outline of the chapter. Write the requested information directly in the spaces provided.

1. What are the four basic steps in billing and collections?

   (1)   (3)

   (2)   (4)

14.1 Patient Financial Responsibility

1. What is the basis of effective patient billing?

Financial Policies

2. List five topics covered in a good practice financial policy.

    (1)   (4)

    (2)   (5)

    (3)

3. How do practices educate patients about the billing and reimbursement process?

Check Processing and Nonsufficient Funds

4. Explain how a NSF check occurs.

5. What are some other terms for a NSF check?

14.2 Working with Patients' Statements

1. What is a patient ledger?

2. What is the day sheet?

3. Define patient statements.

4. What billing steps are taken after the patient encounter?

5. In what three ways is the RA used for billing?

    (1)   (3)

    (2)

6. How does the PMP use this information?

The Content of Statements

7. List the six types of information shown on the patient statement.

    (1)   (4)

    (2)   (5)

    (3)   (6)

Relating Statements to the Practice Management Program

8. How is the ledger card used to create patient statements?

14.3 The Billing Cycle

1. What is cycle billing?

2. How is guarantor billing different from individual statements?

3. What are three advantages of guarantor billing?

    (1)   (3)

    (2)

4. When is guarantor billing typically used?

5. Give an instance when individual billing for various family members would be preferred.

14.4 Organizing for Effective Collections

1. Define collections.

2. List three reasons why patients may not pay their bills.

    (1)   (3)

    (2)

Staff Assignments

3. List three typical job functions of billing and collections.

    (1)   (3)

    (2)

Billing/Collections Manager

4. List three alternate job titles for billing/collections manager.

    (1)   (3)

    (2)

5. List the six typical tasks of the billing/collections manager.

    (1)   (4)

    (2)   (5)

    (3)   (6)

The Patient Account Representative

6. What is the main function of the bookkeeper?

7. What do collections specialists do?

8. What are some incentives used to encourage collections specialists?

Avoiding Opportunities for Fraud

9. How can a practice reduce the chance of employee errors or stealing?

10. Define embezzlement.

11. List three good practices to avoid financial frauds.

(1)   (3)

(2)

14.5 Collection Regulations and Procedures

1. How are collections activities regulated?

2. List the eight guidelines to ensure fair and ethical collections activity.

(1)   (5)

(2)   (6)

(3)   (7)

(4)   (8)

3. How do practice policies fit with these laws?

Procedures

4. What is the purpose of the patient aging report?

5. When does aging begin?

6. What is included in the patient aging report?

7. What are the four categories of patient balances?

(1)   (3)

(2)   (4)

8. How are procedures for collections established?

Collections Letters

9. What is the purpose of the collections letter?

10. What is the general tone of collections letters?

Collections Calls

11. What is the purpose of a collections call?

Collections Call Strategies

12. List six of the general strategies collections specialists can use when placing collections calls.

    (1)   (4)

    (2)   (5)

    (3)   (6)

13. How should the collections specialist handle not reaching the patient but getting another person?

Common Collections Call Scenarios

14. List two probable patient statements and collections specialist responses.

    (1)   (2)

Documentation

15. What is the next step for the billing specialist after ending a phone call?

16. What is the purpose of this documentation?

17. List five common abbreviations and their meanings.

    (1)   (4)

    (2)   (5)

    (3)

14.6 Credit Arrangements and Payment Plans

1. What is a payment plan? What is a benefit of offering a plan?

Equal Credit Opportunity Act

2. What entity enforces the ECOA?

Truth in Lending Act

3. What law governs payment plans that have finance charges, late fees, or more than four payments?

4. How are payment plans that do not have finance charges, late fees, or more than four payments regulated?

Credit Counseling

5. How does credit counseling work for the debtor?

Designing Payment Plans

6. How does the collections specialist design a payment plan?

7. What does a truth in lending form disclose about a payment plan?

Setting Up Prepayment Plans

8. What is a prepayment plan?

9. What is the first step, for insured patients, in creating a prepayment plan?

14.7 Collection Agencies and Credit Reporting

1. Define collection agency.

2. Why would a practice use a collection agency?

3. What is the role of the practice collections specialist when a collection agency is used?

When to Use a Collection Agency

4. At what point is a collection agency usually used for collections?

5. List four reasons a practice would send patient bills to collections agencies before the usual aging point.

(1)   (3)

(2)   (4)

6. Are all debts collected?

Selecting a Collection Agency

7. What is the most important thing to remember in choosing a collection agency?

Types of Collection Agencies

8. What is an advantage of a local agency?

9. What is an advantage of a national agency?

Analyzing the Cost of a Collection Agency

10. Why is choosing the agency with the lowest rate usually not the best method?

Credit Reporting

11. What is credit reporting?

12. What is the function of a credit bureau?

13. What laws regulate the process of credit reporting?

14. What is the purpose of these laws?

Skip Tracing

15. Define skip trace.

Tracing a Debtor

16. What is the first step before beginning a skip trace?

17. When should the collections specialist begin the skip trace process?

18. List four methods used to trace a debtor.

(1)   (3)

(2)   (4)

Professional Skip Tracing Assistance

19. What should be considered before hiring professional skip tracing assistance companies?

Computerized Skip Tracing

20. How can technology help in skip tracing?

21. List three types of computer searches that can be used to trace debtors.

(1)   (3)

(2)

Effective Skip Tracing Calls

22. Are there any laws or guidelines that regulate skip tracing calls?

23. What is a disadvantage of using information obtained from online sources?

Collection Payments Posting

24. What terms must a collection agency follow in transmitting monies to a practice?

14.8 Writing Off Uncollectible Accounts

1. What is an uncollectible account? What is another name for it?

2. What are two areas of concern when dealing with uncollectible accounts?

3. What is a bad debt? What type of accounts might qualify as bad debts?

Common Types of Uncollectible Accounts

4. What is the most common reason accounts become uncollectible?

5. What is the process of a means test? Why is it done?

6. What can be done with accounts of deceased patients that have remaining balances?

7. How can the provider receive payment when a patient files bankruptcy?

8. What is the last step in trying to collect uncollectible accounts?

Dismissing Patients Who Do Not Pay

9. May a physician dismiss a patient?

10. What is the process for dismissing a patient? What information should be documented when dismissing a patient?

Patient Refunds

11. How can patient refunds be handled?

14.9 Record Retention

1. How long and in what form are patients' medical and financial records retained?

2. What is a retention schedule?

3. What are some of the advantages of having a retention schedule?

4. How are decisions about saving financial records generally made?

5. How long should records be retained by HIPAA-covered entities?

KEY TERMS

MATCHING

Match the definition with the correct term from the following word list.

A. bankruptcy	L. guarantor billing
B. bad debt	M. means test
C. collection agency	N. patient aging report
D. collection specialist	O. collection ratio
E. credit bureaus	P. nonsufficient fund (NSF) check
F. credit reporting	Q. patient statements
G. cycle billing	R. payment plan
H. day sheet	S. prepayment plan
I. embezzlement	T. retention schedule
J. Fair and Accurate Credit Transactions Act (FACTA)	U. skip trace
K. Fair Debt Collection Practices Act (FDCPA) of 1977	V. uncollectible account

1. The practice's policy about keeping records, which includes a list of the items from a record, that are retained and for how long.

2. A term used to mean stealing funds.

3. A summary of the financial transactions that occur each day.

4. Printed bills that show the amount each patient owes.

5. A law designed to protect the privacy of credit report information and to guarantee that information supplied by consumer reporting agencies is as accurate as possible.

6. A report designed to determine which patients are overdue on their bills and group them into categories for efficient collection efforts.

7. External agencies that a medical practice can hire to perform specialized collection efforts on difficult debtors.

8. An account that remains unpaid after the practice staff have exhausted all of their collection efforts.

9. The practice of sending one statement to the guarantor of a number of different accounts.

10. The process used to assign patient accounts to a specific time of the month, and to standardize the times when statements will be mailed and payments will be due.

SELF-QUIZ

1. When might a debt be considered uncollectible?

2. Phone calls made for collections purposes are governed by what laws?

3. What is the difference between the patient ledger card and the patient statement?

4. How can the practice help to avoid embezzlement or fraudulent practices?

5. Why is the typical first collection letter more of a reminder letter?

CRITICAL THINKING QUESTIONS

1. Why might patients who are able to pay refuse to pay?

2. Why must the collections specialist document the conversation content of collection calls?

3. How can credit counseling benefit the practice?

4. Why can't a practice create a telephone script for collection calls?

5. Why can't the collections specialist discuss the patient's debt with other persons?

WEB ACTIVITIES

SURFING THE NET

1. Go to AHIMA's website at www.ahima.org.
   A. Using the Search box, search for information on records retention schedules.
      1. How many responses did you get?

      _____

      _____

   2. Select one article to review for information on the current practices in medical records retention.

USING THE WEB WISELY

1. Go to the fair debt collection informational website—www.ftc.gov/bcp/edu/
pubs/consumer/credit/cre18.shtm.

   A. Who maintains this website?

   _____

   _____

   B. What is the purpose of this website?

   _____

   _____

   C. What can you do if you believe a debt collector violated the law?

   _____

   _____

   D. What types of free information can consumers receive to learn about using
   credit?

   _____

   _____

WEB SCAVENGER HUNT

1. Go to FDCPA's website at
www.ftc.gov/bcp/edu/pubs/consumer/credit/cre27.pdf.

   A. When did this act become law?
   B. Who monitors/enforces this law?

APPLYING CONCEPTS

Carlos Nunez owes your practice $157.92; this is the amount not covered by his
insurance plan. The debt is over 60 days past due. Previously you had contacted
Carlos by letter to remind him that he owed this amount and that the insurance
company had paid all they were obligated to pay. In that letter, you encouraged
Carlos to make full payment or contact the office to make payment arrangements.
You received no response to the letter and no payment.

1. Compose the body of a second collection letter to Carlos Nunez.

A new patient, Stanislaw Wisnewski, sought an initial consultation at your practice
for laparoscopic cholesystectomy. He does not have insurance and needs to arrange
a payment plan to pay the surgeon's fees, which total $840. The medical billing
specialist worked with Stan to assure that he would be able to pay; your office does
not charge interest or finance charges for payment plans. Stan stated that he needed
a payment plan/payments that would be less than $60 per month but that he
wanted to pay at least $50 per month.

2. Devise a payment plan for Stan.

Hans and Helga Diethrick and their children, Helmut and Hannah, are patients in your practice. They receive one billing statement for the entire family. Their insurance coverage has a $20 copay. The Diethricks forgot to pay their copays for June; on July 30, a late fee of 1 percent was added to the balance.

3. Complete the Diethrick's ledger card.

Hans Diethrick - guarantor Helga Diethrick – spouse Helmut Diethrick – child Hannah Diethrick - child 939 Allemangel Road Allentown, PA 18105 610-555-9632					Honor Insurance	
Date/Pro		**Charge**		**Payment/Adj**		**Balance**
4/18	OV	Helmut	72.00			
4/18	Copay			Helmut	20.00	
4/30	INS			Insurance		
6/11	OV	Helga	48.00			
6/15	INS			Insurance		
6/23	OV	Hans	96.00			
6/30	INS			Insurance		
7/30	Late Fee		0.40			

Chapter 17 Hospital Billing and Reimbursement

(Note that there are no workbook exercises required for textbook Chapters 15 and 16.)

Learning Outcomes

After studying this chapter, you should be able to:

17.1 Distinguish between inpatient and outpatient hospital services.
17.2 List the major steps relating to hospital billing and reimbursement.
17.3 Contrast coding diagnoses for hospital inpatient cases and for physician office services.
17.4 Explain the coding system used for hospital procedures.
17.5 Discuss the factors that affect the rate that Medicare pays for inpatient services.
17.6 Interpret hospital health care claim forms.

ASSISTED OUTLINING

Directions: Read the chapter through one time. Then go back over the chapter and find the information required to complete the following outline of the chapter. Write the requested information directly in the spaces provided.

1. Why must the medical billing specialist have knowledge of hospital billing?

17.1 Health Care Facilities: Inpatient Versus Outpatient

Inpatient Care

1. What is an inpatient facility?

2. List and describe two types of inpatient facilities.

(1)   (2)

Outpatient or Ambulatory Care

3. Explain outpatient care.

4. List and describe three outpatient services provided in patients' home settings.

(1)   (3)

(2)

Integrated Delivery Systems

5. How does an integrated delivery system work?

17.2 Hospital Billing Cycle

1. How do hospitals usually handle the processing of claims?

2. List several typical hospital departments and their functions in claims processing.

3. What is the typical name of the medical records department in hospitals?

4. List the three steps in a patient's hospital stay.

(1)   (3)

(2)

5. How can hospitals release HIPAA-protected PHI without patient authorization?

Admission

6. What is registration?

7. What is the master patient index?

8. What is contained in the master patient index?

9. How does the HIM department permit access to clinical information?

10. How does the amount of information gathered for hospital admission compare to that gathered for an office visit?

Consent

11. What are the three unique items on a hospital consent form that aren't found on practice consent forms?

(1)   (3)

(2)

Coordination of Benefits

12. What is an MSP account?

Beneficiary Notice of Nonpayment (Medicare)

13. What is the HINN used for?

Pretreatment Patient Payment Collection

14. What types of payments may be collected in advance?

Records of Treatments and Charges During the Hospital Stay

15. Who sets standards for inpatient hospital medical records?

16. What is contained in the hospital inpatient medical record?

17. How are HIPAA requirements usually met by hospitals?

18. What services are patients typically charged for by hospitals?

19. How are patients charged?

20. How are observation services billed?

21. How are physician's fees billed?

Discharge and Billing

22. What is the timeline for filing claims?

23. What is a charge master?

24. What is contained on the master list or charge master for each item?

17.3 Hospital Diagnosis Coding

1. Who does the coding for inpatient hospital stays?

2. What code set is used to code inpatient hospital diagnoses and procedures?

3. What four groups are responsible for the rules concerning hospital diagnosis coding?

(1)   (3)

(2)   (4)

4. How does the coder locate the rules for inpatient versus physician office coding of diagnoses?

5. What is the UHDDS?

Principal Diagnosis and Sequencing

6. How is the concept of principal diagnosis determined for hospital inpatients?

7. How does this differ from coding in medical practices?

Suspected or Unconfirmed Diagnoses

8. How are suspected or unconfirmed conditions coded when patients are admitted for a hospital workup?

Comorbidities and Complications

9. What is a comorbidity?

10. How are comorbidities different from complications?

11. How are these diagnoses noted in the patient's medical record?

12. Why is it important to code comorbidities and complications?

17.4 Hospital Procedure Coding

1. What are the characteristics of a significant procedure?

2. What code set is used to report inpatient procedures?

Code Set Structure

3. Explain the code structure of ICD-10-PCS. How do coders use this format?

4. Where is the ICD-10-PCS code set located? How often is it updated?

Characters

5. What is the format of the codes in ICD-10-PCS?

Coding Procedure and Resources

6. What does the index of the ICD-10-PCS Table list?

7. How do coders proceed after finding the index entry in the ICD-10-PCS?

Principal Procedure

8. What is the principal procedure?

17.5 Payers and Payment Methods

1. What does Medicare A help pay?

Medicare Inpatient Prospective Payment System

Diagnosis-Related Groups

2. What is a DRG?

3. What is the purpose of DRGs?

4. How are groupings created?

5. How are DRGs calculated?

6. What is the case mix index?

7. What is a grouper?

MS-DRGs

8. What is the purpose of a MS-DRG?

Inpatient Prospective Payment System

9. How are most hospital services paid by Medicare?

10. What is the IPPS?

11. What ramifications occur if a patient is held longer than the DRGs allow?

12. How is the DRG rate determined?

Present on Admission Indicator

13. Define *present on admission.*

14. When is the POA indicator used?

Never Events

15. Explain what is meant by *never events.*

Quality Improvement Organizations and Utilization Review

16. What is the original name of QIOs?

17. Who makes up QIOs?

18. What do QIOs do?

19. What is the purpose of QIOs?

20. What are the four possible outcomes of a QIO review?

   (1)   (3)

   (2)   (4)

21. How do QIOs help provide quality care?

Medicare Outpatient Prospective Payment Systems

22. How are outpatient hospital services reimbursed under Medicare?

23. List and explain the three outpatient prospective payment systems being used by Medicare.

   (1)   (3)

   (2)

24. Name two important guidelines that apply to OPPS billing.

(1)   (2)

Other Medicare Prospective Payment Systems

25. Briefly explain how the SNF PPS works.

Private Payers

26. What is an ELOS?

27. How does an ELOS help to reduce costs?

28. How do private payers typically negotiate the fees they pay hospitals?

29. How do PPOs and HMOs typically negotiate the fees they pay hospitals?

17.6 Claims and Follow-up

1. How are Medicare Part A claims electronically submitted by hospitals? What claims are used?

2. If a paper claim is filed, what form must be used?

Health Care Claim Completion

3. What sections requiring data elements are on the 837I or 837P?

UB-04 Claim Form Completion

4. How many data fields are on the UB-04?

Remittance Advice Processing

5. How do hospitals handle RAs?

6. What is the typical turnaround time for claims filed electronically?

Hospital Billing Compliance

7. How are fraud and abuse uncovered in hospital billing?

8. What is MedPar?

9. How is the collected MedPar data used?

10. How can hospitals safeguard against fraud?

KEY TERMS

MULTIPLE CHOICE

Circle the letter of the choice that best matches the definition or answers the question.

1. The condition determined after study as being chiefly responsible for the patient's admission to the hospital.

    A. Principal procedures
    B. Admitting diagnosis
    C. Principal diagnosis
    D. Complication

2. Any person admitted to a hospital for services that require an overnight stay.

    A. Admitting physician
    B. Inpatient
    C. Outpatient
    D. Consultant

3. A payment system used by hospitals that determines the number of hospital days and the hospital services that are reimbursed.

    A. UHDDS
    B. IPPS
    C. OPPS
    D. MS-DRG

4. The paper-based claim form for hospital billing effective March 1, 2007.

    A. UB-92
    B. UB-04
    C. HIPAA 837P
    D. HIPAA 837I

5. The condition identified by the physician at the time of the patient's admission to the hospital.

    A. Principal procedures
    B. Admitting diagnosis
    C. Principal diagnosis
    D. Complication

6. Medicare's system of analyzing conditions and treatments for similar groups of patients that is used to establish Medicare's fees for hospital inpatient services.

    A. UHDDS
    B. IPPS
    C. OPPS
    D. DRG

7. Conditions in addition to the principal diagnosis that the patient had at hospital admission that affect the length of the hospital stay or the course of treatment.

    A. Admitting diagnosis
    B. Principal diagnosis
    C. Complications
    D. Comorbidities

8. Conditions that develop as complications of surgery or other treatments.

    A. Admitting diagnosis
    B. Principal diagnosis
    C. Complications
    D. Comorbidities

9. The main database that identifies patients in a patient register under a unique number.

   A. Case mix index
   B. Master patient index
   C. Charge master
   D. UHDDS

10. This covers all types of health services that do not require an overnight hospital stay.

    A. Hospice care
    B. Home health care
    C. At-home recovery care
    D. Ambulatory care

SELF-QUIZ

1. Why should the office medical billing specialist understand hospital billing?

2. How is an MS-DRG different from a DRG?

3. What is ELOS?

4. What is contained in the master patient index?

5. What happens during the second step of the hospital billing and reimbursement sequence?

CRITICAL THINKING QUESTIONS

1. How is the admitting diagnosis different from the principal diagnosis?

2. How is the approach of the ICD-10-PCS advantageous?

3. How are DRGs different from OPPS?

4. Why would the UB-04 have more form locators or boxes than the CMS-1500?

5. Why is billing a part of the HIM department in most hospitals?

WEB ACTIVITIES

SURFING THE NET

1. Go to the American Hospital Association Clearing House website at www.ahacentraloffice.org/.

2. Click Request Coding Advice. What code sets are available?

   _____

   _____

3. Click on ICD-9-CM. How do you submit a question for review?

   _____

   _____

4. Return to the AHA Central Office home page. What new information is available about the ICD-10?

   _____

   _____

WEB SCAVENGER HUNT

1. Go to the National Uniform Billing Committee website—www.nubc.org.

2. Click on About the NUBC. What is the purpose of this organization?

3. Click on What's New. What is the most current development or release?

APPLYING CONCEPTS

Wilma Mays decided to have elective surgery to replace her left knee due to rheumatoid arthritis. She also has chronic emphysema and Type 2 diabetes. After her three-day hospital stay for the surgery, Wilma was moved to Meadow View Nursing Center. There she received physical therapy, respiratory therapy, monitoring of her blood sugars and insulin dosage, and general nursing care for an additional ten days.

1. To code her hospital stay, what would be the likely principal diagnosis?

2. For billing purposes at Meadow View, is Wilma considered an inpatient or outpatient?

Kamran Ashfar is a Medicare beneficiary. Medicare Part A has a deductible of $952 for hospital days one through sixty and $238 coinsurance per day for days sixty-one to ninety. Kamran had been in the hospital for forty-one days in January, and he is now hospitalized for five days with acute pneumonia. His hospital charges for this visit total $13,652. (Rates based on Medicare Part A 2006 amounts.)

3. What is Kamran's responsibility for his five-day hospital stay?

4. For what amount is Medicare Part A responsible for this second stay?

Kamran is hospitalized once again for a period of nineteen days.

5. What is his responsibility for this third hospital stay?

DRAFT - NOT FOR OFFICIAL USE

HEALTH INSURANCE CLAIM FORM

APPROVED BY NATIONAL UNIFORM CLAIM COMMITTEE (NUCC) 02/12

| | PICA | | | | | | | | PICA | |

1. MEDICARE   MEDICAID   TRICARE   CHAMPVA   GROUP HEALTH PLAN   FECA BLK LUNG   OTHER
(Medicare#) (Medicaid#) (ID#/DoD#) (Member ID#) (ID#) (ID#) (ID#)

1a. INSURED'S I.D. NUMBER   (For Program in Item 1)

2. PATIENT'S NAME (Last Name, First Name, Middle Initial)

3. PATIENT'S BIRTH DATE   SEX
MM   DD   YY   M ☐   F ☐

4. INSURED'S NAME (Last Name, First Name, Middle Initial)

5. PATIENT'S ADDRESS (No., Street)

6. PATIENT RELATIONSHIP TO INSURED
Self ☐ Spouse ☐ Child ☐ Other ☐

7. INSURED'S ADDRESS (No., Street)

CITY   STATE

8. RESERVED FOR NUCC USE

CITY   STATE

ZIP CODE   TELEPHONE (Include Area Code)
(   )

ZIP CODE   TELEPHONE (Include Area Code)
(   )

9. OTHER INSURED'S NAME (Last Name, First Name, Middle Initial)

10. IS PATIENT'S CONDITION RELATED TO:

11. INSURED'S POLICY GROUP OR FECA NUMBER

a. OTHER INSURED'S POLICY OR GROUP NUMBER

a. EMPLOYMENT? (Current or Previous)
☐ YES   ☐ NO

a. INSURED'S DATE OF BIRTH   SEX
MM   DD   YY   M ☐   F ☐

b. RESERVED FOR NUCC USE

b. AUTO ACCIDENT?   PLACE (State)
☐ YES   ☐ NO

b. OTHER CLAIM ID (Designated by NUCC)

c. RESERVED FOR NUCC USE

c. OTHER ACCIDENT?
☐ YES   ☐ NO

c. INSURANCE PLAN NAME OR PROGRAM NAME

d. INSURANCE PLAN NAME OR PROGRAM NAME

10d. CLAIM CODES (Designated by NUCC)

d. IS THERE ANOTHER HEALTH BENEFIT PLAN?
☐ YES   ☐ NO   *If yes*, complete items 9, 9a, and 9d.

READ BACK OF FORM BEFORE COMPLETING & SIGNING THIS FORM.

12. PATIENT'S OR AUTHORIZED PERSON'S SIGNATURE I authorize the release of any medical or other information necessary to process this claim. I also request payment of government benefits either to myself or to the party who accepts assignment below.

SIGNED _____   DATE _____

13. INSURED'S OR AUTHORIZED PERSON'S SIGNATURE I authorize payment of medical benefits to the undersigned physician or supplier for services described below.

SIGNED _____

14. DATE OF CURRENT ILLNESS, INJURY, or PREGNANCY (LMP)
MM   DD   YY   QUAL.

15. OTHER DATE
QUAL.   MM   DD   YY

16. DATES PATIENT UNABLE TO WORK IN CURRENT OCCUPATION
FROM MM   DD   YY   TO MM   DD   YY

17. NAME OF REFERRING PROVIDER OR OTHER SOURCE
17a.
17b. NPI

18. HOSPITALIZATION DATES RELATED TO CURRENT SERVICES
FROM MM   DD   YY   TO MM   DD   YY

19. ADDITIONAL CLAIM INFORMATION (Designated by NUCC)

20. OUTSIDE LAB? $ CHARGES
☐ YES   ☐ NO

21. DIAGNOSIS OR NATURE OF ILLNESS OR INJURY Relate A-L to service line below (24E)   ICD Ind.

A. |_____   B. |_____   C. |_____   D. |_____
E. |_____   F. |_____   G. |_____   H. |_____
I. |_____   J. |_____   K. |_____   L. |_____

22. RESUBMISSION CODE   ORIGINAL REF. NO.

23. PRIOR AUTHORIZATION NUMBER

24. A. DATE(S) OF SERVICE		B. PLACE OF SERVICE	C. EMG	D. PROCEDURES, SERVICES, OR SUPPLIES (Explain Unusual Circumstances)		E. DIAGNOSIS POINTER	F. $ CHARGES	G. DAYS OR UNITS	H. EPSDT Family Plan	I. ID. QUAL.	J. RENDERING PROVIDER ID. #
From MM DD YY	To MM DD YY			CPT/HCPCS	MODIFIER						
1										NPI	
2										NPI	
3										NPI	
4										NPI	
5										NPI	
6										NPI	

25. FEDERAL TAX I.D. NUMBER   SSN EIN ☐ ☐

26. PATIENT'S ACCOUNT NO.

27. ACCEPT ASSIGNMENT? (For govt. claims, see back)
☐ YES   ☐ NO

28. TOTAL CHARGE $

29. AMOUNT PAID $

30. Rsvd for NUCC Use

31. SIGNATURE OF PHYSICIAN OR SUPPLIER INCLUDING DEGREES OR CREDENTIALS
(I certify that the statements on the reverse apply to this bill and are made a part thereof.)

SIGNED _____   DATE _____

32. SERVICE FACILITY LOCATION INFORMATION

a.   b.

33. BILLING PROVIDER INFO & PH # (   )

a.   b.

NUCC Instruction Manual available at: www.nucc.org   *PLEASE PRINT OR TYPE*   OMB APPROVAL PENDING

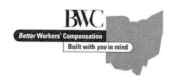

First Report of an Injury, Occupational Disease or Death

Injured worker and injury/disease/death info.

Last name, first name, middle initial			Social Security number	Marital status ☐ Single	Date of birth	
Home mailing address			Sex ☐ Male ☐ Female	☐ Married ☐ Divorced	Number of dependents	
City	State	9-digit ZIP code	Country if different from USA	☐ Separated ☐ Widowed	Department name	

Wage rate
$ _____ Per: ☐ Hour ☐ Month ☐ Week ☐ Year ☐ Other

What days of the week do you usually work?
☐ Sun ☐ Mon ☐ Tues ☐ Wed ☐ Thur ☐ Fri ☐ Sat

Regular work hours
From _____ To _____

Have you been offered or do you expect to receive payment or wages for this claim from anyone other than the Ohio Bureau of Workers' Compensation? ☐ Yes ☐ No If yes, please explain.

Occupation or job title

Employer name

Mailing address (number and street, city or town, state, ZIP code and county)

Location, if different from mailing address

Was the place of accident or exposure on employer's premises? ☐ Yes ☐ No
(If no, give accident location, street address, city, state and ZIP code)

| Date of injury/disease | Time of injury
_____ ☐ a.m. ☐ p.m. | If fatal, give date of death | Time employee
began work _____ ☐ a.m. ☐ p.m. | Date last worked | Date returned to work |
| Date hired | | State where hired | | Date employer notified | |

Description of accident (Describe the sequence of events that directly injured the employee, or caused the disease or death.)

Type of injury/disease and part(s) of body affected (For example: sprain of lower left back)

Benefit application/medical release – I am applying for recognition of my claim under the Ohio Workers' Compensation Act for work-related injuries that I did not purposely inflict. I request payment for compensation and/or medical expenses as allowable. Direct payment(s) to the providers of any medical services are authorized. I understand that I am allowing any provider who attends to, treats or examines me to release all medical, psychological and/or psychiatric information that is causally or historically related to physical or mental injuries relevant to issues necessary to the administration of my workers' compensation claim to the Ohio Bureau of Workers' Compensation, the Industrial Commission of Ohio, the employer listed in this claim, that employer's managed care organization and any authorized representatives. I further authorize the Ohio Rehabilitation Services Commission to release information about my physical, mental, vocational and social conditions that is causally or historically related to physical or mental injuries relevant to issues necessary for the administration of my workers' compensation claim to the aforementioned parties.

| Injured worker signature | Date | E-mail address | Telephone number
( ) | Work number
( ) |

Treatment info.

| Health-care provider name | Telephone number
( ) | Fax number
( ) | Initial treatment date |
| Street address | City | | State | 9-digit ZIP code |

Diagnosis(es): Include ICD code(s)

| Will the incident cause the injured worker to miss eight or more days of work? ☐ Yes ☐ No | Is the injury causally related to the industrial incident? ☐ Yes ☐ No |

| Health-care provider signature | 11-digit BWC provider number | Date |

Employer info.

Employer policy number

Check if ☐ Employer is self-insuring
☐ Injured worker is owner/partner/member of firm

| Telephone number
( ) | Fax number
( ) | E-mail address | Federal ID number | Manual number |

Was employee treated in an emergency room? ☐ Yes ☐ No

Was employee hospitalized overnight as an inpatient? ☐ Yes ☐ No

If treatment was given away from work site, provide the facility name, street address, city, state and ZIP code

☐ **Certification** - The employer certifies that the facts in this application are correct and valid.

☐ **Rejection** - The employer rejects the validity of this claim for the reason(s) listed below:

For self-insuring employers only
☐ **Clarification** - The employer clarifies and allows the claim for the condition(s) below:
☐ **Medical only** ☐ **Lost time**

| Employer signature and title | Date | OSHA case number |

BWC-1101 (Rev. 8/2005)

FROI-1 (Combines C-1, C-2, C-3, C-6, C-50, OD-1, OD-1-22)

This form meets **OSHA 301** requirements